A
Thousand Miracles
Every Day

A Selection of Stories that
Shaped the Mission and History of
Adventist Hospitals

By
Jane Allen Quevedo
Forward by Mardian J. Blair

TEACH Services, Inc.
Brushton, New York

Copyright © 2003 TEACH Services, Inc.
ISBN 1-57258-241-3
Library of Congress Catalog Card No. 2002109733

Published by

TEACH Services, Inc.
www.tsibooks.com

ACKNOWLEDGMENTS

For his vision to produce this collection of stories, his
wise counsel and overall direction of the project, and
his commitment to see it finished:

Mardian J. Blair

❧

For their careful review of the manuscript and helpful suggestions:

*Wally Coe, Pat Benton, Frank Dupper, William Murrill,
Ray and Virginia Pelton, Benjamin Reaves, Don and Doris Roth,
Royce and Elaine Thompson, Rita Waterman
and many, many others*

❧

For sharing their experiences, letters, tapes and other documents:

Dozens of Kind and Helpful People Around the World

❧

For designing the cover:

Mark Bond

❧

For the cover photo:

Paradise Valley Hospital, Ed Guthero and Stan Sinclair

❧

For the corporate sponsorship that made this book possible:

*Adventist Health System
111 North Orlando Avenue
Winter Park, FL 32789*

CONTENTS

Foreword vii

Introduction x

Part 1: THE EARLY YEARS

Vision, Verandas and Divine Providence 3

Where Adventist Healthcare Began in the West—
  St. Helena Hospital 6

Colorado Mountain Resort—Boulder Memorial Hospital 12

Northwest Pioneers—Portland Adventist Medical Center 15

Retreat for the Sick and Tired—Walla Walla General Hospital 20

On the Shore of Spot Pond—Boston Regional Medical Center 23

Wheel of Providence Turns—Paradise Valley Hospital 29

Burden's Twenty-dollar Deal—
  Glendale Adventist Medical Center 33

Not for Any Common Purpose—
  Loma Linda University Medical Center 38

When David Paulson Prayed—Hinsdale Hospital 45

Healthy Spot on God's Footstool—
  Washington Adventist Hospital 53

Rocky Venture on the Cumberland—
  Tennessee Christian Medical Center 58

Parmele's $9,000 Success Story—Florida Hospital 64

The Lord Would be Pleased—Park Ridge Hospital 70

Training Center in the City—White Memorial Medical Center 74

Mother D's Promise—Riverside Sanitarium and Hospital 80

Influence of a Surgeon's Prayer—Takoma Adventist Hospital 84

Forty-five Cent Refund—Porter Adventist Hospital 89

CONTENTS

Part 2: OVERSEAS GROWTH

Diamond Mines, Dispensaries and Dedication 97

AFRICA—Diamonds in the Rough 99

AFRICA—The Parsons in Angola 105

AFRICA—Mission to Uganda 110

ASIA—Blessings, Bombs, and Tiger Tales 148

ASIA—For the Love of China 118

ASIA—A Thousand Miracles Every Day 124

ASIA—Land of Morning Calm 130

ASIA—Opportunities in India 137

ASIA—Bygone Days of Burma 141

ASIA—Setting Sail for Siam 143

ASIA—War's End Closes Vietnam Hospital 148

AUSTRALIA—Land Down Under 153

INTER-AMERICA—Slow Growth South of the Border 160

INTER-AMERICA—Sweet Beginnings in Puerto Rico 163

EUROPE—Bathtubs, Elastics and a King's Villa 166

SOUTH AMERICA—From Argentina to the Amazon 171

Part 3: POST-WORLD WAR II

Bucket Brigades, Quilt Raffles and Multi-million-dollar Gifts 183

Resort Reborn—Florida Hospital Heartland Medical Center..........185

Pearl in Paradise—Feather River Hospital 188

$52,000 for a Pair of Socks—North York Branson Hospital..........193

Golden Days in Sierra Foothills—Sonora Community Hospital 198

Battle Creek Revisited—Battle Creek Adventist Hospital..............201

More Than a Hospital for Navajos—Monument Valley Hospital ..204

Homegrown in America's Heartland—
Shawnee Mission Medical Center............................207

Right Place at the Right Time—
Hanford Community Medical Center........................211

Hawaiians Wait for Hospital—Castle Medical Center 214

Built on Excellence—Kettering Medical Center.............................216

Every Dollar Counts—Memorial Hospital......................................225

Lessons in Hometown Fund Raising—
    Hackettstown Community Hospital 231

Serving Cheese and Salmon Country—
    Tillamook County General Hospital 235

Mission to Appalachia—Jellico Community Hospital....................239

Dentist Honors His Parents—
    Huguley Memorial Medical Center...249

Miracles of Ukiah—Ukiah Valley Medical Center 252

Shuffleboard Courts and Fitness Trails—
    East Pasco Medical Center...255

Fountain Pen Legacy—Florida Hospital Waterman 261

Part 4: APPENDIX

A: Why SDA Hospitals?..265

B: Chronology 269

FOREWORD

In early 1999 I addressed a group of healthcare and church leaders at a Conference on Mission sponsored by Adventist Health System in Orlando, Florida. It was my final presentation to this group prior to my retirement January 1, 2000, and I shared some stories I had heard during my career in Adventist healthcare.

One involved Dr. Ralph Waddell, who established Bangkok Adventist Hospital in the 1930s. I mentioned Dr. Theodore Flaiz and his tiger-hunting adventures in India, and I told about the 45-cent refund to a Denver businessman who later built the Porter Sanitarium and Hospital. I also shared Nurse Gertrude Green's wartime experiences in China in the 1930s and 1940s.

I also recalled my early days in Adventist healthcare. I told about my boss A.C. Larson at Hinsdale Hospital, and how our conversations sometimes turned to the early days of Adventist hospitals. This was an important part of my education as an up-and-coming healthcare executive in the Seventh-day Adventist Church. It taught me about the history and culture of the organization to which I would devote my professional life.

Most of the people in my audience that day in 1999 had never heard these stories, but their comments afterward seemed to be more than polite. I was impressed with the value of publishing a selection of stories related to the history, development and culture of Adventist hospitals.

While individual organizations publish their own histories from time to time, I believe there is a need for a single volume that brings together many of these stories. It can serve as a resource not only for leaders of the denomination's healthcare organizations, but also for church members, community leaders, healthcare professionals, students and many others.

I invited Jane Allen Quevedo, communication director at Adventist Health System from 1985 to 1995, to gather the information and write this book. She brings to the project more than 25 years of writing, editing and teaching experience in Adventist organizations, including New England Memorial Hospital, the General Conference of Seventh-day Adventists, Far Eastern Division headquarters in Singapore, Faith For Today, Pacific Union College and Adventist Health System/Sunbelt. Upon my retirement, Adventist Health System continued to support her efforts and provide the valuable corporate sponsorship that made this book possible.

We chose to focus on Adventist healthcare developments subsequent to the first facility in Battle Creek because a wealth of information on that organization already exists. A brief review of the Battle Creek story introduces the first section of this book and establishes a background for the stories that follow. Of course, Battle Creek's influence is evident throughout the early years of Adventist healthcare, and even in some of the post-World War II hospitals.

We further established boundaries by limiting coverage to hospitals in operation in 2000, with a few exceptions. Throughout the 19th and 20th centuries Adventists started scores of healthcare facilities around the world. While many are now closed, some were important in Adventist healthcare history and thus we included them.

Our search for stories and information took many routes, beginning with the *1999 Seventh-day Adventist Yearbook*, which provided a list of about 150 hospitals. Then we found facts, history and an overview of each hospital in the *Seventh-day Adventist Encyclopedia* (*The Seventh-day Adventist Bible Commentary* CD-ROM, Hagerstown, Maryland: Review and Herald Publishing Association, 1995, and *Seventh-day Adventist Encyclopedia*, revised edition, Washington, D.C.: Review and Herald Publishing Association, 1976.) Hospital websites provided additional details.

The search moved to books, brochures, articles, letters, documents, unpublished manuscripts and tape recordings. Finally a number of personal interviews provided details, memories and dozens of stories. In a few cases we found limited sources beyond the *Seventh-day Adventist Encyclopedia*. Other sources are listed at the end of each chapter.

Organization of the book fell naturally into three eras: The Early Years, Overseas Growth and Post-World War II. Although it was not the intent to produce an all-inclusive history, this book does provide a broad historical overview. No attempt was made to include every hospital or to treat all hospitals equally. The objective was to gather human-interest stories, and present them within the context of each hospital's history.

While sharing her experiences as a missionary nurse in China and Thailand, Gertrude Green (1907–2002) mentioned that if she were to write a book, she would call it *A Thousand Miracles Every Day*. The significance of her title became profoundly clear as this book manuscript developed. The stories here reveal the vision, sacrifice and dedication of those who pioneered Adventist medical work around the world. With Green's permission, and in her honor and memory, we adopted her title.

The stories of Adventist healthcare are filled with examples of divine providence and intervention: Green tells of a company of soldiers that retreats when met by a "huge army" coming toward them—an army that she believes was sent by God. Many years earlier, Dr. David Paulson repeatedly receives unexpected gifts of money that arrive at the exact time they are needed to build Hinsdale Hospital. In South America, a minister approaches a woman at a train station and as a result finds a cure for the disease called "savage fire." Indeed, some things are difficult to explain from a human perspective.

History clearly reminds us how much healthcare has changed since the mid-1800s. I certainly would not wish to return to the days when young nurses carried buckets of hot water up three flights of stairs, employees had no paid vacation days and retirement plan, or hospital administrators put liens on the homes of elderly patients who could not pay their bills. At the same time, history helps keep our mission in focus.

An organization that loses sight of its history risks losing its purpose. With time, the early stories become lost, forgotten, or so changed that they bear little resemblance to the actual experience. Memories fail, books go out of print, pioneers die. We hope this book helps preserve many of the stories which not only reflect the heritage of Adventist healthcare, but most importantly, illustrate God's blessing and providential leading in the lives of people who see healthcare as the human expression of the healing ministry of Christ.

Mardian J. Blair
President Emeritus
Adventist Health System

INTRODUCTION

At the height of its popularity, the world-famous Battle Creek Sanitarium attracted the likes of Henry Ford, Thomas Edison, J.C. Penney, Clara Barton, George Bernard Shaw, John D. Rockefeller, Jr., Dale Carnegie and Amelia Earhart. They and hundreds of others came to Battle Creek to recuperate from the stress and intemperance of their busy lives. Here they would get hydrotherapy treatments and massages, participate in recreational and exercise activities, and dine on sometimes-experimental dishes designed for the most health-conscious.

Certainly, one of the sanitarium's biggest attractions was its medical director, Dr. John Harvey Kellogg, a skillful surgeon, advocate of vegetarianism and proponent of the natural laws of health. Kellogg joined the Western Health Reform Institute about nine years after it opened, renamed it Battle Creek Medical and Surgical Sanitarium, and developed it into a world-famous center. At its prime in the 1920s, it could accommodate 1,500 guests.

The Battle Creek Sanitarium was founded on the concept that healthcare was vital to Seventh-day Adventists' mission to relieve human suffering. Ellen White, author, speaker and visionary accepted by the church as divinely inspired, believed in the interrelationship of physical, mental and spiritual well-being. She promoted a rational approach to health, emphasizing exercise, rest, wholesome diet, fresh air, sunshine, water, abstinence from harmful substances and trust in God.

The well-documented Battle Creek story represents the first chapter in the history of Adventist healthcare. The Seventh-day Adventist Church had already established its headquarters and a publishing house in Battle Creek when it opened the Western Health Reform Institute in 1866, and soon afterward it would open Battle Creek College.

These organizations produced many nurses and other medical missionaries who could teach, preach and give simple health treatments. Wherever they went, the Adventists from Battle Creek took healthcare with them—lecturing at evangelistic meetings, operating treatment rooms and sanitariums, or dispensing medicines at overseas mission stations. For a short time the church even operated a medical school at Battle Creek, graduating several physicians who helped establish some of the facilities that are the anchors of Adventist healthcare today.

Thus begins the next chapter of Adventist healthcare, and the first major section of this book. Nearly 20 of today's Adventist hospitals opened their doors during Mrs. White's lifetime (1827–1915). In the United States these include St. Helena Hospital, Portland Adventist Medical Center, Walla Walla General Hospital, Paradise Valley Hospital, Glendale Adventist Medical Center, Loma Linda University Medical Center, Hinsdale Hospital, Washington Adventist Hospital, Tennessee Christian Medical Center, Florida Hospital, Park Ridge Hospital, and White Memorial Medical Center. The early overseas facilities include Sydney Adventist Hospital, River Plate Sanitarium and Hospital, Malamulo Hospital, Lake Geneva Sanitarium, and Simla Sanitarium and Hospital.

Adventist healthcare's third era emerges after the denomination established the College of Medical Evangelists in Loma Linda, California, in 1909. While early missionaries had operated treatment rooms and dispensaries, and even established overseas sanitariums, the years between 1915 and 1945 saw a tremendous increase in the number of overseas facilities. In the United States, only two Adventist hospitals in operation today were established during this time—Takoma Adventist Hospital in 1928, and Porter Adventist Hospital in 1930.

The end of World War II ushered in the era of the Adventist community hospital. New medicines and technologies, insurance plans, Medicare and other advances changed healthcare forever. Sanitarium programs featuring lectures, recreation and extended "vacations" soon became history. The early health centers shed the "sanitarium" part of their names as their business shifted to acute care.

By this time Adventists were known for operating a special kind of hospital where caregivers recognized the importance of treating the whole person, and gave extraordinary care. Communities across the United States invited the church to help them build and operate their hospitals.

As medical science brought technological advances and capabilities, Adventist hospitals added programs and services to meet the needs and expectations of the ever-increasing number of people they served. Today's tertiary-care hospitals greatly expand the church's healthcare ministry in terms of quality and service.

A Thousand Miracles Every Day traces the history of Adventist healthcare up to its current era, the development of health systems. In the late 1960s, leaders such as Don Welch at Florida Hospital and Erwin Remboldt at Glendale Adventist Hospital, as well as certain church leaders, recognized the need to strengthen individual facilities to survive the coming changes and competition of newly organized for-profit hospital corporations.

With the system organization, the church's hospitals could benefit from economies of scale by centralizing programs such as purchasing, information systems and malpractice insurance. They also created a pool of management expertise to oversee all the denomination's hospitals, not just the big ones. And, they provided vehicles for acquiring other hospitals that could not compete as stand-alone facilities. The large systems and medical centers continue to have a distinct advantage in attracting smaller hospitals and systems seeking to align with strong parent organizations. The consolidation begun in the 1970s continues today.

Over the years, thousands of men and women helped develop Adventist healthcare around the world—John Burden in California and Australia; Percy Magan at Madison and Loma Linda; Harry Miller in China; Leo and Jessie Halliwell in Brazil; Robert and Della Habinecht in Argentina; Roy and Mabel Parsons in Angola; Daniel and Lauretta Kress in England and Australia; Nellie Druillard in Tennessee, George Nelson at Kettering, Ohio; and many others.

In spite of hardships, these pioneers remained steadfast in their mission. Some sold their homes to build hospitals. They took on personal debt and worked long hours, sometimes without pay. Some were ostracized, persecuted and even killed. Some lost loved ones to disease and accidents. Some gave up personal ambitions and lucrative positions to serve in places where success depended upon their own ingenuity and the grace of God. More than one miracle was performed in a small mission hospital where a lone physician worked in an improvised facility with inadequate equipment.

No avenue of service by the Seventh-day Adventist Church touches more lives than its healthcare work. It has created an international awareness of the church, united Adventists in a common mission with local communities, and strengthened their ministry in those communities.

A Thousand Miracles Every Day records some of the human-interest stories related to the development of Adventist hospitals from the late 1800s to the beginning of the 21st century. It chronicles the vision, sacrifice, dedication and overriding hand of divine providence in their histories. As a ministry, Adventist healthcare must always recognize its place in God's plan to care for those who are sick and hurting. In this context it continues to be a story of miracles—more than a thousand every day.

Part 1

The Early Years

Chapter 1

Vision, Verandas and Divine Providence

Pattern Established

Every Adventist healthcare organization traces its heritage to Battle Creek, Michigan, where the young Seventh-day Adventist Church established the Western Health Reform Institute in 1866. Typically the history of an early Adventist hospital begins with a description of a Victorian structure surrounded by broad verandas and spacious lawns where guests relaxed and enjoyed outdoor activities in the fresh air and sunshine. A collection of photographs might show patients arriving at a sanitarium in a horse-drawn buggy, nurses in white starched uniforms giving hydrotherapy treatments, and stern-faced physicians posing next to the latest medical invention of the early 1900s. The narrative describing early days at "The San" likely discusses the visionary leadership of Ellen White, and the innovative Dr. John Harvey Kellogg, who devoted 68 years of his life to helping people live healthfully.

While Mrs. White and Dr. Kellogg were key figures in the history of the Battle Creek Sanitarium, another White and another Kellogg figured prominently in the pioneer effort, too. Mrs. White's husband, James, and the doctor's father, J. P. Kellogg, were among those who bought company stocks to begin the institute. Kellogg, father of 11 children, operated a broom factory, and for many years generously supported the fledgling church.

From the beginning James White supported the health center. In the early days, when it appeared that it would not succeed, he took over and rescued it from failure. A few years before this, he had suffered ill health due largely to overwork and poor diet. He went to a New York facility specializing in water treatments. While making some improvement, he did not fully recover until he changed his diet and followed his wife's advice to add some physical and mental activity to his daily program. White's experience gave added impetus to his wife's counsel that the Seventh-day Adventist Church should establish a health ministry as "the right arm" of its gospel ministry.

Under White's administration, the institute's sagging bottom line began improving. However, to be a successful enterprise, it needed

3

qualified physicians. Over the years the Whites had watched the Kellogg children and were especially taken with young John Harvey. They encouraged him to study medicine and return to Battle Creek, and even paid some of his school expenses. Kellogg studied at the Trall's Hygieo-Therapeutic College in New Jersey, the University of Michigan and Bellevue Hospital Medical College in New York. Then he returned to Battle Creek, and at age 24 was appointed medical superintendent.

Kellogg was an energetic, enthusiastic, inventive and persuasive personality with big ideas. Traveling around the world, he preached the gospel of health and promoted his ideas on "biologic living." He invented, among other things, peanut butter, cornflakes, exercise equipment and even a mechanical horse for President Calvin Coolidge.

He studied surgery in Europe under some of the world's leading physicians. It is reported that he performed more than 22,000 operations. Dr. Dunbar Smith, who served at the Battle Creek hospital in the 1950s, had opportunity to examine some of Kellogg's patients and found the surgery scars barely visible.

Even after Kellogg joined the sanitarium, the need for qualified physicians was a problem. To help alleviate the situation, promising students were selected to pursue medicine at secular universities. Often, however, they returned to Battle Creek with ideas that didn't fit squarely with the philosophy of the sanitarium. Around 1891 a plan was developed for students to share a home in Ann Arbor while studying at the University of Michigan. This provided them an Adventist Christian environment while they studied at the university.

The class included David Paulson, future founder of Hinsdale Hospital near Chicago, Edgar Caro, future medical director of the forerunner of Sydney Adventist Hospital in Australia, and Daniel and Lauretta Kress, who later served in England, Australia, New Zealand and at Washington Sanitarium and Hospital in Takoma Park, Maryland.

Unsatisfied with the arrangement of educating prospective doctors, the Battle Creek Sanitarium board voted to begin a medical school under Kellogg's leadership. American Medical Missionary College opened in 1895, with the main campus in Battle Creek, and the clinical division in Chicago, directed by Paulson.

The medical school, free clinics and other expansion severely drained the denomination's finances. Church leaders wished to keep the sanitarium small, adding other facilities as opportunities arose and money became available. Among other things, Kellogg and the church also disagreed over admission policies to the medical school, points of doctrine, and ultimately ownership of the sanitarium. Among the biggest controversies was the rebuilding of the facility after fire destroyed it in 1902.

Kellogg ignored the counsel he had been given to construct a single building, not more than five stories high and 450 feet in length. Instead, he built a huge structure featuring marble pillars and five acres of marble mosaic floors—reported to be the best-equipped facility of its kind in the world.

Unable to work with Kellogg, and wishing to avoid centralization of their work, church leaders focused their attention elsewhere. In 1903 they moved their headquarters to Washington, D.C., and began looking for a place for a medical school. They found a number of failed healthcare facilities and resorts at bargain-basement prices in Southern California, and purchased one near San Bernardino called Loma Linda. In 1906 they opened a school, which would become the College of Medical Evangelists, today's Loma Linda University.

Many members of the staff and faculty joined the California school. Although enrollment at American Medical Missionary College declined and the school closed in 1910, Kellogg operated the Battle Creek Sanitarium until his death in 1943. While he and the church never officially reconciled, certainly Kellogg and the Battle Creek Sanitarium played important roles in establishing the medical work of the Seventh-day Adventist Church. As the following pages reveal, their influence was felt for many years in hospitals, dispensaries, clinics and treatment rooms all around the world.

SOURCES

Robinson, D.E., *The Story of Our Health Message*, Nashville, Tennessee: Southern Publishing Association, 1956.

Schaefer, Richard A., *Legacy: Daring to Care*, Loma Linda, California: Legacy Publishing Association, 1995.

Schwarz, Richard W., *John Harvey Kellogg, M.D.*, Nashville, Tennessee: Southern Publishing Association, 1970.

Smith, Dunbar W., M.D., *The Travels, Triumphs and Vicissitudes of Dunbar W. Smith, M.D.*, Loma Linda, California: Dunbar W. Smith, M.D., 1994.

Chapter 2

Where Adventist Healthcare Began in the West

St. Helena Hospital
Established 1878

Another Dr. Kellogg

Before the first Adventist health center opened in Battle Creek, or the first Seventh-day Adventist missionary sailed the Atlantic, or John Harvey Kellogg entered medical school, Merritt Gardner Kellogg trekked across the United States in an oxcart. Arriving in San Francisco in 1859, the eldest Kellogg brother and his family are thought to be the first Seventh-day Adventists in California.

Kellogg worked as a carpenter to pay the bills, but his real passions were sharing his faith and establishing church congregations. Seeing a great need for health education and medical care, he returned to the East in 1867 to complete a six-month medical course, which in those days qualified him to use the title "Doctor."

Others joined Kellogg in California, and by the mid-1870s Adventists in the state numbered around 500, or about six percent of the entire denomination's membership. While looking for a place to build a church in the Napa Valley, leaders found an ideal location for a health center in St. Helena. Three years later Kellogg helped establish the facility and served as its first medical director.

Believing that his work in California would be more effective if he had some medical training, Kellogg moved to New Jersey in 1867 and enrolled at Trall's Hygieo-Therapeutic College. Before returning to the West Coast, he persuaded two others to join him, J.N. Loughborough and D.T. Bourdeau. This threesome worked together for some time, with the ministers preaching the gospel and the doctor giving health lectures.

High Success Rate

When a smallpox epidemic broke out near Santa Rosa in 1870, Kellogg and Loughborough stopped their public meetings to tend to the sick. People were impressed by the doctor's successful treatment with water therapy and healthy diet. It is reported that about 10 of every 11 patients recovered under his care, compared to only one in five by another physician using popular drug treatments of the day.

Kellogg later settled in the Napa Valley, a few miles south of St. Helena. There he continued his medical practice while working closely with the ministers. The number of Adventists in California grew steadily. Among the converts were two men who made it possible to build the first major Adventist health center on the West Coast. Today St. Helena Hospital is the oldest Seventh-day Adventist healthcare center in the world.

Loughborough, president of the newly organized California Conference of Seventh-day Adventists, had helped establish the Battle Creek health center, and hoped someday to start a similar facility in Northern California. He and one of his associates, I.D. Van Horn, were in St. Helena in 1874, working on plans to build a church. While looking for potential sites, Van Horn found an attractive hillside property overlooking the valley. It had a spring, and he thought it was an ideal place for a health center. The property belonged to William Pratt, a retired bricklayer and recent convert to the Adventist faith.

However, nothing happened with that idea until sometime later when Kellogg was caring for a patient. The doctor and the patient's husband, A.B. Atwood, talked of the need for a medical facility and soon they were making plans. Atwood came up with $1,000, Kellogg gave $1,000 in labor, and Pratt donated 10 acres of his hillside property.

Reporting in the church magazine *Signs of the Times* (November 22, 1877), Kellogg proclaimed, "The location is all that could be desired…. The climate, location and surroundings are not second to any other locality in California for the recovery and preservation of health."

Backbreaking Work

Among the stockholders was John Morrison of Santa Rosa, who received $200 worth of stock in payment for a team of horses used to haul lumber. Construction of a two-story frame building began in 1878, with the foundation bricks made of clay from the local hillsides, and baked in kilns in Pratt's yard.

The 13-bed Rural Health Retreat in St. Helena opened in June 1878. Ellen White spoke at the dedication, declaring, "...the very surroundings exert an influence in calling us to higher and purer lives." Within a week, every bed was occupied and tents were pitched in the yard to house employees and patient overflow. In fact, some early guests preferred to stay in tents to fully enjoy the mountain air.

With the health center completed, Kellogg moved to Los Angeles in 1879. Four years later, he sailed to the South Pacific on the second voyage of the mission vessel *Pitcairn*. He served several years in the islands of Tonga and later in Australia.

Another significant figure in early Adventist healthcare, John Burden, joined St. Helena Sanitarium as business manager in 1891. At that time the facility was reportedly the largest of its kind on the West Coast. It even had branches in San Francisco, Sacramento and Eureka, California, and Honolulu, Hawaii. Burden was later instrumental in developing three major Adventist healthcare facilities in Southern California—Paradise Valley, Glendale and Loma Linda—as well as the Sydney Sanitarium in Australia.

St. Helena Sanitarium (renamed in 1890) opened one of the first schools of nursing in California, and was the first to graduate a male nurse. Interestingly, male nurses in those days did not perform such bedside tasks as taking a patient's temperature and pulse. The men chopped wood, delivered specimen jars and set up cots for the night shift. According to 1928 graduate Olin Bray, male nurses gave hydrotherapy treatments during the day and were assigned "cot duty" with alcoholic and psychiatric patients at night.

Sweet Concoctions

While studies and work occupied much of their time, the male student nurses found time for some enterprising ventures such as making their own root beer. "They filled disposable glass intravenous flasks with their 'brew' and frequently shared it with the girls. Root beer floats concocted from the boys' stock and cafeteria ice cream were a favorite for many years."—PAT BENTON

The thriving health retreat spawned a little community known as Sanitarium, with a post office that opened in 1901. In the aftermath of the 1906 San Francisco earthquake, many fled to this mountain community. Again tents were put to good use as temporary housing.

An historical transcript describing the St. Helena Sanitarium in 1939 offers a glimpse of daily life typical of Adventist health centers in the

1930s and 1940s. While the facility provided acute-care medical, surgical and maternity services, it also offered the traditional sanitarium programs featuring hydrotherapy, massage, nutrition, physical and occupational therapy and other preventative medicine programs. At St. Helena, the sanitarium section was completely separate from the acute-care facility.

Sanitarium guests arriving by car were met by pages who escorted them across the veranda and inside to the registration desk. A hand-operated elevator transported guests upstairs to the comfortably furnished rooms, some having writing desks and vanities for their convenience.

There were probably fresh flowers in the room, too, because employees used to gather wildflowers from the Napa Valley. In addition, guests were permitted to cut flowers from the sanitarium gardens where they were usually assigned to work.

Life at the San

Each day began with reveille and the raising of the flag at sunrise. Guests were expected to be on the roof at 7 a.m. where a physical therapist led them in morning exercises—complete with live piano accompaniment. Other activities included croquet, tennis, archery and darts.

Guests who were able took their meals in the dining room, along with staff members, and visitors from all over California's North Bay Area. A dining room hostess seated the guests, who selected their meals from a menu and were served by waiters. St. Helena Sanitarium and Hospital served vegetarian food exclusively from 1915 until 1984. (The collection of birds, fish and deer on the hospital campus were strictly for the guests' visual enjoyment, and never appeared on their dinner plates.)

An intercom system throughout the hospital kept patients aware of various activities, such as the evening parlor program or twice-a-day band concerts performed by hospital employees.

While medical science and healthcare have changed dramatically since the 1930s, the world's oldest Adventist health center continues to help hundreds of people through its comprehensive hospital-based wellness programs. The St. Helena Center for Health provides 19 residential rooms for individuals participating in lifestyle enhancement programs such as diet and wellness, smoking cessation, weight management and alcohol/chemical dependency recovery. Nearly 125 years after the St. Helena Hospital was founded, this tranquil, private setting overlooking the Napa Valley remains a perfect backdrop for learning the principles of healthful living.

The hospital's physical plant developed over the years as healthcare changed and the staff endeavored to meet patient needs. The original structure was replaced in 1968. However, during the next few years St. Helena Hospital faced one of the most critical times in its history and was in danger of closing in the early 1970s. Looking for a way to turn around finances and meet the community's needs, St. Helena took a bold step by starting a cardiology program, including open-heart surgery.

Heartfelt Turnaround

A group of physicians pooled funds in 1972 to equip a cardiovascular catheterization lab, making St. Helena Hospital the first in California's North Bay Area to perform coronary angiograms. Dr. Charles Tam used to fly from Southern California on Sundays to perform angiograms with Dr. Wilson White. Finally Tam and his physician brother Wilfred moved to St. Helena in 1974. Working with White, they created the first cardiac surgery team and program in the area. Before emergency coronary angiograms and coronary artery bypass procedures were even options at most hospitals, they had become standard treatments for heart attacks at St. Helena Hospital.

With the development of a strong, loyal medical staff any idea of closing the program was put to rest as St. Helena Hospital grew into the region's leader in cardiac care. In 1981 the first coronary angioplasty was performed here, and in 1999 the cardiac team performed its 7,000th open-heart surgery. A second state-of-the-art cardiac catheterization laboratory opened in 2001.

While it met some big challenges in its long history, the hospital managed to weather the storms of change, and still remains faithful to its mission of health and healing.

SOURCES

"A Century of Progress 1878–1978: St. Helena Hospital and Health Center Celebrates 100 Years," 1978.

Benton, Pat, "From Hydrotherapy to Heart Surgery," *Pacific Union Recorder*, August 5, 1991.

Johns, Warren L., and Richard H. Utt, editors, *The Vision Bold*, Washington, D.C.: Review and Herald Publishing Association, 1977.

"St. Helena Sanitarium and Hospital: Established 1878," undated.

"Sanitarium Dedication, Open House Sunday, *St. Helena Star*, May 9, 1968.

"Transcription of Historical Tape," undated.

"Where the Ministry of Healing Takes Place," *Pacific Union Recorder*, June 6, 1978.

Interview: Erwin Remboldt.

Chapter 3

Colorado Mountain Resort

Boulder Memorial Hospital
1893–1989

Where Do the "Lungers" Go?

My grandfather arrived in Denver in the late 1890s looking for a tuberculosis cure. He did not have the name or address of a TB facility, but his neighbors in North Dakota had told him there was one in Colorado. So, he bought a train ticket and figured he would find the place after he got there. As soon as he arrived, he started asking, "Where do the 'lungers' go?"

"Go right back to Union Station and take the train to Boulder," one man told him. "The 'Advents' have built a place right up against the mountains and they will take good care of you."

After about two months of sunshine, exercise, improved diet, plenty of water and hydrotherapy treatments at the Colorado Sanitarium, Granddad was well on his way to recovery. However, he had no money to pay his bill of about one dollar a day. The sanitarium allowed him to pay off the debt by working as an elevator operator.

In those days employees were expected to attend morning and evening devotions, and my grandfather faithfully attended each meeting. He acquired a Bible and soon became very interested in the Adventist faith and lifestyle. When time came to leave Boulder, he wondered how his family would respond to his new way of life.

My grandmother immediately remarked how well Grandfather looked. She also noticed that on Saturday he did no more than his essential farm chores. He spent much of the day reading, and she likely enjoyed having a quiet day with him and the children. At the same time, she knew a lot of the farm work had been left undone while he was gone. It was not like him to rest when there was work to be done.

"I'm surprised that you are not working on the farm today," she said.

"I, too, am surprised to see you resting today," he said, having noticed that she was not doing her usual Saturday house cleaning.

"Well, I don't know exactly how to tell you," she began as she reached for a book. "A salesman came through while you were gone, and I bought this book from him. After reading it, I now observe the Sabbath from sunset Friday to sunset Saturday."

On examination, they realized she had purchased a Seventh-day Adventist book. Shortly after this, both of my grandparents joined an Adventist church. In 1901 they moved to Colorado and in 1906 my grandfather was instrumental in establishing Campion Academy in Loveland. Through the years they continued to depend on the Colorado (Boulder) Sanitarium for their occasional healthcare needs. —DR. ROBERT HORNER

The gold rush of 1858 and 1859 enticed thousands of fortune-seekers to Colorado, but the real population boom came several decades later, with the flood of tuberculosis patients known as "lungers." By the 1920s more than half of Denver's population was attributed to the TB treatment facilities.

In nearby Boulder, Adventists had opened the Colorado Sanitarium in 1893 sometime after a retired minister had visited the area, and persuaded Dr. John Harvey Kellogg to start a health program there.

The cool mountain setting of the Boulder-Colorado Sanitarium, as it was named in 1905, attracted people wishing to escape the steamy summer weather of Texas and other southern states. For outdoor recreation, they enjoyed horseback riding and mountain climbing, as well as nature walks. The Boulder facility followed the blueprint of other early Adventist sanitariums, offering scientific medical care while promoting the concepts of wellness and natural healing.

Dr. Kate Lindsay was among the first physicians on the sanitarium's closed medical staff, and served there for about 20 years. However, H.A. Green, director of the facility from 1910 to 1937, is the physician most closely linked with the early days of the Boulder San. In fact, for many years it was known as "Dr. Green's Sanitarium." It was renamed Boulder Memorial Hospital in 1962.

Dramatic changes came to this hospital and the church's other healthcare facilities with the transition from the sanitarium era to the age of acute-care hospitals. The Boulder hospital bridged the old with the new by building upon its long-established hydrotherapy program. It developed a state-of-the art physical medicine and rehabilitation department that ranked among the best in Colorado.

However, with a changing marketplace, increased competition and resulting financial losses, the Boulder facility was sold in 1989. A 50-bed

13

replacement facility called Avista Adventist Hospital opened in 1990 in the growing community of Louisville, about six miles from Boulder. Louisville is a thriving young community near the University of Colorado and home to several high-technology industries. Approximately half of the Avista employees formerly worked at Boulder Memorial Hospital.

SOURCES

Briggs, Bill, "Denver Stands Tall Among Healthiest Cities," *Denver Post*, April 15, 2001.

Interviews and Notes: Dr. Robert Horner and Ron Sackett.

Chapter 4

Northwest Pioneers

Portland Adventist Medical Center
Established 1893

Sanitarium for Nervous Diseases

Dr. Louis Belknap was robbed while traveling through San Francisco and arrived in Portland, Oregon, nearly penniless. The student of Dr. John Harvey Kellogg had traveled from Battle Creek to the "Wild West" in 1893 to begin a healthcare venture. Although Adventists had established churches in Oregon as early as the 1870s, they had not established any medical work.

Pastor T.H. Starbuck loaned the doctor some money to get his work started. Belknap rented an eight-room house and set up a six-bed "sanitarium for nervous diseases," specializing in hydrotherapy and water-cure treatments.

With financial help from local church members, in 1895 Belknap set up the Portland Sanitarium in the Reed Mansion, a large ornate house with room for 20 patients, a surgical ward, office, kitchen and dining room. With the house came a stable that was remodeled for treatment rooms and a nurses' dormitory.

After the Belknaps moved to California in 1896, the Adventist church, through the International Medical Missionary and Benevolent Association, took over the sanitarium. With a two-year nurses' training program and the Portland Sanitarium Health Food Company established in 1897, the Portland San charted its course as the church's flagship facility in the Northwest.

By 1902 the sanitarium had outgrown the Reed Mansion. Several acres were purchased on Mt. Tabor, where a four-story, 75-bed facility was built for $50,000. This bright red wooden structure with broad verandas could be easily identified against the green hillside. With no improved roads leading to the site, a steam train from Portland brought patients to within a few blocks of the San.

Dr. William Holden, a highly regarded physician and surgeon, joined the medical staff in 1903. Although sanitarium care continued at the Mt. Tabor facility for some time, Holden's surgical skills attracted patients and helped the hospital to grow into a modern medical center. By 1919 surgery represented about half of the sanitarium's business.

A Family Legacy

Holden and members of his family have served continuously on Portland's medical staff since 1903. Holden was on staff until his death in 1955, serving as medical director from 1910 to 1920, and again from 1924 to 1943, for a total of 29 years. Dr. William Rippy, Holden's son-in-law, later served on the staff, followed by his grandson, Dr. William (Bill) Rippy. Today Holden's great-grandson, Dr. Wesley Rippy, continues the family legacy and mission of Christian healthcare in Oregon.

తా

Along with Holden, Ralph Nelson, business manager/administrator from 1918 to 1955, helped lay a strong foundation for what the San would become. In 1944 he was the first Adventist hospital leader to be named administrator. During his tenure he saw the hospital through many changes and at least two major crises—paying off the debt from the 1903 construction and rebuilding the sanitarium in the early 1920s.

Within a year of paying off the 1903 construction debt in 1919, Mount Tabor was annexed to Portland, and the city fire department condemned the top two floors of the wooden structure. The last patient was admitted August 31, 1920, and the sanitarium closed September 21. Wasting no time, Nelson rallied the community and church and raised $90,000 to build a 50-bed replacement facility on the Mt. Tabor site. The new hospital opened none too soon. Even before painters and plasterers completed their work, Holden performed an emergency appendectomy in the new operating room. Various expansion projects followed from 1924 through the early 1960s. With the exception of the 1964 expansion, all were funded primarily from operating surplus.

By the late 1960s, the Portland San again needed to expand. Not only was the Mt. Tabor site too small, but it was also on the side of an extinct volcano and the soil was not suitable for building a large hospital. Learning of the availability of the 232-acre Glendoveer Golf Course, hospital leaders bought it for $3 million. While they planned to use part of the land for the hospital and develop the remainder into a championship golf course and driving range, the community adamantly opposed the idea.

Mardian Blair became administrator in 1970, and set out to gain public support for the Glendoveer project—even assigning the management team to distribute brochures and solicit signatures in support of it.

"It was a tough job," recalls Don Ammon, president of Adventist Health, and former executive vice president at Portland. "I remember day after day, evening after evening, going door to door around Glendoveer to see if I could get signatures."

The matter was divisive, placing some people in the difficult situation of balancing loyalties between the hospital and community. Among them was Dr. Eldon Snow, whose home backed up to the golf course. While he supported the hospital's position in whatever way he could, he had to be careful not to raise the ire of his neighbors.

In addition to the community relations issue, there was a long certificate-of-need and land-use process. Although the hospital had received a certificate of need for its new facility, after a two-and-one-half-year battle, the county planning commission reversed an earlier decision and denied the land-use permit. Before it was all over, proponents and opponents had their "day in court."

"It was like a trial in city hall," recalls Ammon. "There were testimonies, cross examination and expert witnesses."

In the end, the county paid the hospital the $3 million it had paid for the property, and today continues to operate the golf course.

About the time the county denied permission to build a hospital on the Glendoveer property, a 40-acre site near Portland Adventist Academy became available—a prime location with easy access to the proposed Interstate 205. The hospital bought the land and broke ground in 1974. A physicians' office building opened in 1976, and the new Adventist Medical Center opened in 1977. Additional professional buildings have been built in recent years.

The Mt. Tabor hospital was eventually converted into a convalescent facility, and the oldest portion of the original 1922 sanitarium was demolished in 1980.

A determined effort was made in the early 1970s to recruit specialty physicians to the staff. The Northwest Medical Foundation was established, initially to recruit physicians for Portland and two sister organizations, Walla Walla General Hospital in Walla Walla, Washington, and Tillamook County General Hospital in Tillamook, Oregon. Northwest Medical Foundation eventually developed into a major component of today's Adventist Health, parent organization for Adventist healthcare in the church's North Pacific and Pacific Union Conferences.

In order to attract specialists to the staff, the hospital needed a strong primary-care base to generate referrals. One solution was to develop group practice outpatient clinics through another organization called VertiCare Corporation. Thanks to a $500,000 grant from the Robert Wood Johnson Foundation, VertiCare opened several primary-care clinics. Although these were not financially successful, they did help expand the hospital's service area, says Larry Dodds, former CEO of Portland Adventist Medical Center, and presently senior vice president of Adventist Health. While some of the first clinics have closed and new ones have opened, some of the original clinics remain in operation today.

When the grant ended in 1979, the clinics were turned into private-practice offices, and the hospital did not operate physician practices again until 1985. By this time the major hospitals in Portland had coalesced into distinct systems, which gave them an advantage in obtaining managed-care contracts. Having no partner hospitals in the Portland market, the Adventist hospital aligned with its physicians and purchased some physician practices.

"We just became more powerful because we had the physicians and hospital working together. Nobody else did," explains Dodds, "We were able to sit at the table with healthcare payers and negotiate."

Although the model of physician/hospital relationship continually changes as the market and healthcare industry change, Dodds says Portland Adventist Medical Center's success is clearly attributable to medical staff development. Some of the physicians recruited in the early 1970s have remained at Portland and are now beginning to retire. Today's 302-bed medical center is a testimony to their service, as well as the contribution they and many others have made in the name of Christian healthcare in Portland, Oregon.

"One of the hospital's strengths is its spiritual mission," says Dodds. "We were able through the years to recruit people who had a genuine interest in creating a supportive environment where mission and spiritual care were paramount. The nurses and other staff have created a unique difference because of the continued emphasis on spiritual care for years and years."

Prayer Made All the Difference

I had an appointment with a former patient's daughter one day. Her mother had been hospitalized for about three weeks and then died. I was a little nervous, thinking most family members don't make an appointment to see a CEO unless there is a problem of some kind. When I opened my office door the woman shoved an envelope into my hand.

"You need to read this," she said.

I sat down and began to read the letter. It was very positive about the care our staff had given her mother. She mentioned names of nurses and others who had cared for her. I thanked the woman, and said I'd like to share her letter with our employees.

"Tell me, over the three weeks that your mother was in our hospital, did anything special stand out that I could tell them?" I asked.

"Yes, one morning I left my mother's room for a few minutes. She was in a coma and other family members were around. When I came back to the room some nurses were attending to Mom, so I stopped at the door. Then I realized one of them was praying. That really helped me at a difficult time. I'll never forget it." —LARRY DODDS

SOURCES

Judd, Wayne, tape recorded interviews with Don Ammon, Frank Dupper and Erwin Remboldt, 1998.

"Portland Adventist Through The Years," 1993.

Interviews: Larry Dodds and Monty Knittel.

Chapter 5

Retreat for the Sick and Tired

Walla Walla General Hospital
Established 1899

A Pleasant Place in Springtime

"The Walla Walla Sanitarium is located at College Place in the beautiful Walla Walla Valley which is one of the finest fruit sections of the United States. In the spring time one can stand on the veranda and look out on the celebrated Blalock Fruit Ranch of thirteen hundred acres, four hundred of which are large bearing trees. When these are in bloom one looks upon a veritable sea of flowers. It is hard to find a more pleasant place in the spring than surrounds the sanitarium." —1906 BROCHURE

Dr. Isaac Dunlap and his wife, Maggie, a nurse, returned to the Walla Walla Valley in 1899 after completing their studies in Battle Creek. In fact, the doctor had graduated with the first class from American Medical Missionary College. Their mission in the rural Washington community located in the "Valley of Many Waters" was the beginning of today's Walla Walla General Hospital.

Seventh-day Adventists had opened a college in Walla Walla in 1892, and in 1899 the Dunlaps started treatment rooms in the basement of the administration building. In addition to providing hydrotherapy and other treatments, they also offered a medical missionary course, which 12 young people completed in 1900.

Three years later the Dunlaps built a house on College Avenue that served as both their residence and a sanitarium for the college. Along with conventional treatments of the day, they encouraged a balanced program of physical exercise and rest along with sunshine, fresh air, a vegetarian diet and trust in God. They planted a large garden where patients could relax and work outdoors.

For a while the doctor split his time between Walla Walla and the Mountain View Sanitarium in Spokane. Unfortunately, the Spokane structure burned in 1904. Rather than rebuild, the undamaged equipment was moved to Walla Walla and the two operations merged.

The newly formed Walla Walla Sanitarium rented space in a college dormitory for a couple of years before moving again in 1907. The College Place public schoolhouse was moved onto the college campus, hoisted on jacks and a new floor added underneath. This structure was expanded three times, and by the 1920s had been transformed into a two-story facility with white pillars and wide verandas. The advertising slogan of that era was "A Retreat for the Sick and Tired."

With the purchase of a bankrupt hospital on Bonsella Street for $75,000, the San moved off the college campus in 1931. The facility was fully equipped with the latest in medical supplies. It also came with an unpaid grocery bill for $20,000.

The sanitarium struggled through the 1930s by trimming salaries and personnel, and cutting costs where possible. Telephones, for example, were limited to those deemed most essential. Business picked up in the 1940s and by the end of 1950 plans were underway to expand. Other expansion projects followed, but by the 1970s hospital leaders decided to build an entirely new campus rather than add again to the Bonsella building.

Ron Sackett moved to Walla Walla from White Memorial Medical Center in Los Angeles in 1973. Knowing little about Walla Walla—except that his in-laws lived there—he accepted the position sight unseen.

"When I got to Walla Walla, I found the average age of the medical staff was about 67. There was only $60,000 in the bank and a new hospital to be built," he recalls. His first tasks were to develop the medical staff and raise money for a new hospital.

If that wasn't enough, he soon realized that the proposed location for the new hospital—on the grounds of the local Veteran's Administration—was unsatisfactory. It had no population, no physicians' offices and no convenient transportation. Accompanied by other Adventist healthcare officials, Sackett took an airplane ride over the area to determine the concentration of population and physicians' offices.

"We found a piece of land that had good access to all that. Then we went to see if we could buy it," says Sackett.

Saved for This Purpose

Fearing that the owners might raise their price, the group did not reveal who they were or how they wanted to use the 18-acre property. Disappointed to learn that the land was not for sale, they agreed to make it a matter of prayer. A few days later they went back to the owners, this time explaining their plans to build a hospital. The owners said they had been saving the property for just such a project.

In order to save on construction costs, the hospital found nearby Walla Walla College to be an invaluable resource. The engineering department faculty, headed by Professor Fred Bennett, assisted in planning and designing the facility. As a result, the hospital was built at a cost of $4.5 million—only $55 per square foot. The grand opening on July 10, 1977, drew a crowd of about 3,000.

Today Walla Walla General Hospital is a 72-bed facility with a level III trauma-certified emergency center serving an area of nearly 60,000 residents. While many changes have occurred over the years, the hospital continues the mission begun more than a century ago by a young couple from Battle Creek.

SOURCES

Benton, Pat Horning, "Staying Well Is Better than Getting Well," *North Pacific Union Gleaner*, May 21, 1999.

Benton, Pat Horning, "Celebrating a Century of Caring and Sharing," *A Century of Care*, Walla Walla General Hospital, June 6, 1999.

Chappel, Heather, "History Script," 1999.

Interview: Ron Sackett.

Chapter 6

On the Shore of Spot Pond

Boston Regional Medical Center
1899–1999

Soft-spoken Strong Leader

"*Dr. Ruble never scolded anyone publicly. If he saw a minor rule infraction, he would stare at you without saying a word; but the message was clear. If a severe reprimand was in order—whether you were a doctor, supervisor or maid—he would call you to his office. There he would remind you of the rules, regulations and principles under which the hospital functioned. You were expected to abide by them. He always spoke in a soft voice. A second warning was usually not necessary.*

"*One day his secretary called to tell me that Dr. Ruble wanted to see me in his office. At first I was a little frightened. I put off going to his office for at least three hours, trying to figure out a way to defend myself. But defend against what? The concern that came to mind most frequently was that I was dating a student nurse. One of the strictest rules of the nurses' training program was that student nurses could not date staff doctors. It could mean suspension for the nurse and loss of privileges for the doctor.*

"*I finally got up the courage to see Dr. Ruble. His secretary greeted me with a smile. If only Dr. Ruble could do the same, I thought. She escorted me into his office. He, too, greeted me with a smile, but it was a faint smile.*

"*Then he said, 'I'm glad you like to bring your patients to this hospital.' He kept staring at me through his thick glasses. I thought his next statement would be, 'If you want to continue sending your patients here…'*

"*But he didn't say that. He talked about the hospital. He talked about patients in general. He talked mostly, however, about the Depression and the problems it presented. As he spoke in his usual soft voice, I could feel my fears melt away. I remember his last words: 'My hopes and dreams are that some day this wooden building will be replaced by a beautiful, modern hospital.'*" —DR. ARTHUR TAURO

❧

The close of the 20th century marked the end of an era of Adventist healthcare in the Boston suburb of Stoneham. Known over the years as New England Sanitarium, New England Sanitarium and Hospital, New England Memorial Hospital and finally Boston Regional Medical Center, this facility was the church's anchor hospital in the northeastern corner of the United States for 100 years.

Established as the eastern branch of the Battle Creek Sanitarium, the New England San began in 1895 in a dormitory at South Lancaster Academy about 40 miles north of Boston. By 1901 it was attracting more than 500 patients a year, making it necessary to house them in private homes.

As early as the late 1890s, Ellen White was advising the church to find a larger place for the New England Sanitarium. She directed them to a site on the shore of Spot Pond in Melrose. (The address was later changed to Stoneham.) Two men traveled from Battle Creek to Massachusetts where they found a large wooden building known as The Hotel Langwood on the shore of Spot Pond. However, it was not for sale—not at any price.

Interestingly, many of the hotel's patrons came for more than a night's lodging. It had a thriving gambling business—complete with a cockfighting pit in the cellar and a hidden gambling room.

Mrs. White insisted that a second attempt be made to buy the property. This time the owners agreed to sell, but at a price much too high for the church. On a third visit in 1902, the Adventists discovered that fire had destroyed a large part of the building. At last they succeeded in making a deal—$39,000 for 45 acres, plus buildings and furniture. According to the *Seventh-day Adventist Encyclopedia*, the property was valued at $98,000.

Meanwhile, in South Lancaster the sanitarium had become an annoyance to local residents, notably the influential Thayer family who enjoyed the area's birds, trees and flowers. The story is told that one day Mrs. Thayer went to a window to enjoy the pleasant view around her home and became upset by the scene of wheelchairs, patients and student nurses cluttering the area. She insisted that her husband do something about them.

Thayer, who owned the railroad to Boston, offered to buy the building and move it. The sanitarium leaders accepted his offer and tore down the facility, leaving only the school in South Lancaster. As promised, Thayer moved the lumber, portions of the building, and patients to the Langwood property. The 23-bed sanitarium officially opened its permanent home in 1902. Although an 18-bed wing was added later, a fire on New Year's Day 1905 damaged 25 rooms and destroyed other facilities, including the stables and horses.

The facility was rebuilt after the fire, and over the years various expansion projects gradually increased the size of the plant. One of the most interesting projects involved dismantling a Shaker village in New Hampshire to build the 26-bed Browning Memorial addition and another building known as Glenhurst.

Return to Nature

"Our great lawns, wooded with grand oaks, stately elms, graceful maples and fragrant pines stretch down to the very edge of a beautiful lake.

"We have our own dairy, bakery and farm which ensure our guests the best service and the purest and freshest foods.

"It is our fundamental belief that health is a legitimate harvest of a correct daily life and obedience to the laws of one's being.

"The real purpose of this institution is to return to nature as far as possible and to follow simplicity and naturalness without riding any hobby or following any fad." —1909 SANITARIUM ADVERTISEMENT

The New England San was typical of Adventist health centers of the early 1900s. Most patients were not acutely ill. Except for surgical and obstetrical cases, most came for hydrotherapy treatments, a healthy diet, lectures and other sanitarium activities.

Outdoor activities included pitching horseshoes, riding horses, playing tennis and croquet, or playing golf on the sanitarium's nine-hole course. On one occasion, someone used a horse-drawn mower to trim the lawn, and the horses' iron shoes made deep holes in the grass. The problem was quickly corrected by fitting the horses with specially designed leather boots.

Dr. Wells Allen Ruble, medical director from 1929 to 1943, was one of the New England Sanitarium's most influential personalities. A graduate of American Medical Missionary College in Battle Creek, he had played a prominent role in the early days of the College of Medical Evangelists and had been a missionary in South Africa and Europe.

Alice Smith, retired nurse administrator and educator who was born in the Langwood building and completed nurses' training at New England, remembers Ruble as a godly man.

"He had chapel every morning, and we frequently sang one of Florence Nightingale's favorite hymns, 'The Son of God Goes Forth to

War,'" she recalls. "In those worship meetings, he clearly outlined the goals of the organization."

Whenever patient census was low, the doctor made it a matter of prayer at the employees' daily worship services, and it seemed that the census always improved. He also talked with the employees about fear and illness, and the effect the caregiver's attitude had on patients during wartime.

While Dr. Ruble tended to administrative and mission-related matters, English-born May Ruble devoted her attention to the San's cultural life—sometimes in a style that amused young student nurses.

In the dining room, Mrs. Ruble made an effort to ensure that meals—which often included fruits and vegetables from the San's orchard and garden—were relaxing and pleasant. Either she or a callboy announced mealtimes by tapping musical chimes on each patient floor.

"Probies"—student nurses in their first six months of schooling—served in the dining room as part of their training. Smith recalls that Mrs. Ruble was very particular about how they handled the water glasses.

"She told us to always pick them up by the bottom, never by the top."

Smith also recalls that she and some of her rather vivacious classmates were asked not to sit together in the dining room because they laughed too much.

Roll Out the Music

Music was a part of sanitarium life. Occasionally a band or orchestra was invited to perform on the front lawn. On one of these occasions Mrs. Ruble hurriedly came up to one of the nurses' stations.

"What is that number they are playing?" she asked. "I know it. It's by one of the great masters."

The nurses recognized that even though the band had deliberately slowed the tempo, the tune they were playing was clearly "The Beer Barrel Polka."

∾

The New England Sanitarium School of Nursing graduated 750 nurses during its 63-year history, many of whom devoted their careers to Adventist healthcare. One was a young woman from Macon, Georgia, who graduated in 1940 and would serve as associate director of the medical department of the General Conference of Seventh-day Adventists from 1960 to 1977.

Mazie Herin was one of the school's first students from the South. She had learned about it from an advertisement on the back of a church paper.

"There was this gorgeous picture of a lake, and I thought it would be nice to attend school near a lake where I could go swimming, fishing and boating," says Herin. "When I got there, I found it was just a reservoir. My dreams of playing in Spot Pond at the New England Sanitarium were never realized."

The first months of nursing school were called "probie days," and the students looked forward to January when they would learn whether they could continue the program. Each was called to the nursing director's office where Edith Strand, director of the school, enjoyed giving a personal touch to each announcement. For example, she asked Herin if she thought she'd be able to pin up her hair for capping.

She told Smith, "I've heard very good reports about your nursing. I've also heard your voice from fifth floor down to second."

Black Stocking Debate

In the 1930s student nurses wore black stockings in winter and white in summer. Herin disliked the black stockings and decided to take up the matter with Strand.

"Why do we have to wear these black stockings?" she asked.

"It's because of the snow," the director replied.

"All we have to do is cross the road to the tunnel to get to the hospital. We don't even get out in the snow."

Strand wasn't persuaded, but the young woman from Georgia had the last word.

"I get tired of people looking and commenting about legs. The men just see legs!"

Student nurses provided free labor seven days a week. After working all morning, and attending classes all afternoon, they went back to work in the evening. This allowed little time for study. Herin vowed that if she ever had anything to do with nursing schools, she would change that practice—a promise she kept years later at the Florida Sanitarium and Hospital.

The New England Sanitarium expanded several times during the last half of its 100-year history. A 50-bed wing added in 1951 was named in Ruble's honor. The West Wing built in 1969 replaced the main building constructed in 1906. Most of the funds for the $3.5 million West Wing came from the Stoneham Rotary Club and local community.

Renamed Boston Regional Medical Center in 1995, after suffering severe financial difficulties, the hospital closed in 1999.

SOURCES

Knott, Bill, "Grieving for the 'San,'" *Adventist Review*, April 22, 1999.

Tauro, Arthur L., M.D., *A History of New England Memorial Hospital*, Revised Second Edition, 1999.

Interviews: Ann Gibson, Gertrude Green, Mazie Herin, Ray Pelton and Alice Smith.

Chapter 7

Wheel of Providence Turns

Paradise Valley Hospital
Established 1904

Deep Search for Water

"What are you going to do, Brother Hamilton?" Ellen White queried of the well driller, who had dug to about 80 feet in search of water on the drought-plagued property that she had helped purchase in National City, California.

Salem Hamilton responded with another question. "Did the Lord tell you to buy this property?"

"Yes," she said, assuring him that not once, but three times the Lord had shown her this property.

Harrison's reply was forever etched in the history of Paradise Valley Hospital: "The Lord would not give us an elephant without providing water for it to drink."

&

In 1901 Ellen White told Dr. T.S. Whitelock of her interest in beginning a sanitarium in the San Diego area. A nationwide financial depression in the 1890s had left a number of resort properties in Southern California available at attractive prices, and Mrs. White believed these offered excellent opportunities for the church. (See Chapters 8 and 9 on Glendale Adventist Medical Center and Loma Linda University Medical Center.)

Some time following this discussion, Whitelock, a graduate of American Medical Missionary College in Battle Creek, and a Sophie Johnson operated a successful treatment center in San Diego. It was one of the doctor's patients who told him of an abandoned sanitarium in nearby National City.

Dr. Anna Mary Longshore Potts, a woman of Quaker heritage, had developed the 20-acre property, which consisted of a main building, residence, stable and cottage for employees. Soon after the facility opened in 1888, the region experienced a prolonged and severe drought. Wells all over the area dried up, once-profitable businesses closed, and people moved from the area. Potts closed the sanitarium and turned it over to her uncle, Dr. T.H. Harrison of New York. He put it on the market for $28,000.

By the time Mrs. White visited the site, it had been abandoned for about 14 years. Most of the trees and shrubs had died, and bats occupied the main building. Nevertheless, she said she had never seen a building better adapted for a sanitarium. The main structure with about 50 rooms had a large veranda where patients could relax and enjoy the view.

Not everybody was as eager to start a health facility in National City as were Whitelock and Mrs. White. The church's small Southern California Conference with fewer than 1,200 members was already $40,000 in debt. Further, the denomination's world headquarters, the General Conference of Seventh-day Adventists, was financially strapped in large part because of its early medical work, and had no intention of incurring more debt for healthcare facilities.

Whitelock managed to negotiate Harrison down to $8,000, but it still remained out of the question for the Southern California Conference. Meanwhile, Mrs. White and her friend Josephine Gotzian, a generous contributor to other church organizations, each agreed to come up with $2,000, not knowing where they might get the remaining $4,000.

Still keenly interested in the sanitarium, Whitelock, as well as other potential buyers, frequently visited the Potts property. On one of these occasions in January 1904, the doctor struck up a conversation with a woman at the site. When he introduced himself, she seemed surprised.

"You are the very person I'm looking for," she said.

It seems that Harrison had sent her to get an offer from Whitelock. She suggested $6,000. The doctor had only $4,000. His offer was wired to Harrison, who immediately accepted it. Even though within a matter of hours another party offered him $6,000, Harrison stuck to his agreement with Whitlock.

Without Further Delay

"A special opportunity came to us in the form of a property a few miles south of San Diego known as the Potts Sanitarium. The Lord had manifestly prepared the way for us to begin sanitarium work at this point; and when the wheel of providence turned in our favor, and the property came within our reach, we felt as if we must act without further delay, notwithstanding the hesitancy of brethren in responsibility, who should have been quick to discern the advantages of this place as a center for medical missionary work." —ELLEN WHITE

☞

With assistance from a family who paid the back taxes and purchased eight additional acres, Paradise Valley Sanitarium started on an investment of less than $6,000. A stock company was formed to raise funds with the idea that the Southern California Conference would eventually take it over.

The first order of business was to repair the run-down plant, and most important, find a water source. E.R. Palmer, who had been in Australia when Mrs. White lived there, managed the new venture in National City. Although repairs were extensive, Palmer spent as little money as possible. It is told that he mended a shingle roof with small pieces of tin cans. He also found a good deal on some high-quality furniture made of bird's-eye maple.

From the beginning, founders of Paradise Valley Sanitarium knew they must find water, and hopes must have dimmed as the drought continued through the summer of 1904. At Mrs. White's recommendation, Palmer hired a well digger from Nebraska. Digging the well turned into a long and slow process, but when workers finally reached water, they found a gully-washer. In fact, water poured in so quickly they did not stop to gather their tools.

Guests began arriving before repairs were completed, and on opening day the sanitarium already had 20 patients. Although Paradise Valley attracted a large clientele, the first couple of years were difficult. Repeated attempts failed for the Southern California Conference to take over the sanitarium.

To further complicate matters, the opening of two other Southern California facilities in Glendale and Loma Linda greatly hindered recruitment at Paradise Valley. Employees preferred to work at these new church-owned sanitariums. Mrs. White personally solicited funds for the sanitarium and published a brochure detailing God's providential leading in the purchase of the property. Paradise Valley was also among the facilities to benefit from the sale of her book, *Ministry of Healing*.

Frequent management changes and medical staff turnover hurt the sanitarium's reputation in the early years. However, through persistence and hard work, Paradise Valley finally showed a profit in 1910, and ownership transferred to the Southern California Conference in 1912.

John Burden, who had served at St. Helena and Sydney and had been instrumental in obtaining the properties at Glendale and Loma Linda, managed Paradise Valley Sanitarium from 1916 to 1924, and again from 1925 to 1934.

The Lord Supplies Our Need

A.C. Larson led Paradise Valley Sanitarium through many challenges during his administration from 1934 to 1944. The years of the Great Depression and World War II required unusual ways of meeting the financial requirements to run a hospital. For example, Larson told about the time he needed $3,000 for payroll. Finally he called his key leaders and asked them to join him in his office. They were kneeling in prayer when Larson's secretary entered the room and tapped him on the shoulder. She handed him a note saying that a woman had just given the hospital a check for $3,000.

Though growth continued through the 1950s, the 1960s marked big changes for Paradise Valley with the opening of a new 150-bed replacement hospital in 1966. Also, the last nursing class graduated in 1967.

Programs and facilities continued to be added as the hospital grew to meet the needs of the diverse communities in the San Diego area. Today Paradise Valley Hospital is a modern 237-bed facility offering a full range of inpatient and outpatient services.

SOURCES

Johns, Warren L., and Richard H. Utt, editors. *The Vision Bold,* Washington, D.C.: Review and Herald Publishing Association, 1977.

Judd, Wayne R., and Jonathan M. Butler, editors. *Thirsty Elephant: The Story of Paradise Valley Hospital*, National City, California: Paradise Valley Hospital, 1994.

White, Ellen G., *The Paradise Valley Sanitarium*, Mountain View, Calif.: Pacific Press Publishing Association, 1909.

Interview: Mardian Blair.

Chapter 8

Burden's Twenty-dollar Deal

Glendale Adventist Medical Center
Established 1905

A Grand Place

"I grew up in the Glendale San community during the 1930s, a few years after the hospital relocated to Chevy Chase Drive. It was majestic with its parlor, dining room, solarium and manicured landscape. The zoo was fascinating with monkeys, bears, deer and other animals. The huge powerhouse was impressive. To the families from Michigan it was a poor substitute for the Battle Creek Sanitarium, but we could not imagine anything grander than the new Glendale Sanitarium and Hospital."
—DR. ROBERT HORNER

After moving ahead without church backing at Paradise Valley, Ellen White next began pressing for the purchase of another property. Still convinced that the church risked missing some real bargains following the depression of the 1890s, she urged leaders to build another sanitarium in Southern California. Finally, growing impatient over the delay, she asked her friend John Burden to go to Los Angeles to look at available properties. She knew his work well at St. Helena Sanitarium in California and Sydney Sanitarium in Australia. Burden trusted White implicitly. When faced with a difficult decision of whether to heed her counsel or follow instruction from church leaders, Burden could be counted on to side with her.

He found a number of likely locations in the Los Angeles area, the most promising being the 75-room Glendale Hotel. Located on a five-acre plot and built at a cost of $60,000, the facility had never opened as a hotel. Although it housed a school for a short time, it stood empty when Burden found it on the market for $26,000 in 1904. The quiet country location with about 500 residents would be ideal for a sanitarium. There was even an electric car line running past the property, providing easy access to Los Angeles. While Burden knew it was a bargain, he also knew church leaders would not agree to buy it. At last he reasoned that if the realtor could whittle the price to $15,000, he would consider it a sign from the Lord and move ahead with the purchase.

Realtor Leslie Brand was probably the most notable figure in the early development of the Glendale area. Burden told him of the plan to build a facility similar to the famous Battle Creek Sanitarium, and when he said the church didn't have much money, Brand dropped the price to $12,500. The story is told that Burden immediately handed him a $20 bill, having no idea where he would get the rest of the money. Brand also helped remove a stipulation that prohibited the use of the property for a sanitarium.

While a $20 bill may have sealed the deal, Burden still needed the down payment. Not surprisingly, the church constituency voted against the purchase. At that time the Southern California Conference of Seventh-day Adventists had little more than 1,000 members and around $40,000 in debt. Fortunately, Conference President Clarence Santee shared Burden's conviction that the opportunity to buy the hotel at that price likely would never come again. Since the church did not have money, he and Burden personally advanced the down payment, not knowing how the balance would be paid.

From her home in Northern California, Mrs. White wrote to church leaders urging them to buy the Glendale property. Santee read her letter at a meeting of conference delegates, who immediately pledged $5,200. With $1,000 advances from two other church members, the conference made a $4,500 cash payment, put the rest in a bank, and paid the balance over the next three years.

Burden became manager, and immediately set to work with a group of volunteers, who had Glendale's first medical facility mopped, scrubbed, sterilized, painted and open for business in August 1905. Soon guests were enjoying the place an early brochure described as "the fruit-laden valleys of the 'Land of Sunshine and Flowers.'"

To meet staffing needs, the sanitarium began training nurses—with a strict regimen based on the principle of all work, no play and low pay. Student nurses received six cents an hour during their first year and 10 cents in their second year. Nothing was to interfere with sleep, studies or work—certainly not parties, recreation or courtships. By the time the nursing program transferred to Pacific Union College in 1967, the Glendale Adventist Hospital had graduated 1,282 nurses.

As Glendale's population boomed to nearly 30,000 by the early 1920s, the sanitarium outgrew its original facility. The property was sold for $250,000 dollars, of which $50,000 was used to buy 30 acres for a replacement hospital. Construction began immediately—on a hill of apricot groves between the San Rafael foothills and the Sierra Madres.

Unfortunately, costs escalated to more than a million dollars. With a major reorganization that put Burden in charge again, the new sanitarium opened in March 1924. The debt, however, would not be paid off until the late 1930s.

Expansion continued and new services were added over the next several decades, keeping pace with the growing city. Two key figures during this time were George Nelson, administrator from 1947 to 1959, and Erwin Remboldt, administrator from 1960 to 1973. During Nelson's administration the hospital celebrated its 50th anniversary with the opening of a new wing, bringing the total patient beds to 292.

By the early 1960s most of the Glendale San's business was acute-care, with only a few long-term sanitarium patients. The hospital was the largest in the city and enjoyed an excellent reputation. While it was rapidly moving away from the sanitarium business, the facility continued to maintain some features from the by-gone days, such as an aviary and a small zoo with several monkeys. The zoo finally gave way to new construction when a 60-bed mental health unit opened in 1963—built in part with Hill-Burton funding.

Keep Up or Close Down

For many years, the church had provided small subsidies to its hospitals, and contributed to major building programs. These funds were extremely limited and eventually abolished. The Hill-Burton Act of 1946 made federal funds available to build or rebuild healthcare facilities, but some questioned whether accepting these funds crossed the line on the separation of church and state. At the same time, many Adventist hospitals were aging and in need of renovation or replacement. With new technology and services coming into the industry, church leaders faced the reality that the hospitals must keep up or close down. Glendale was one of the church's first hospitals to receive Hill-Burton funding. Hospital and church leaders made sure the contract had a provision allowing the hospital to discriminate on religious issues.

"The attorney put it in there, and the audit was based on that contract," says Frank Dupper, retired president of Adventist Health, who served at Glendale Adventist Hospital from 1964 to 1974.

Medicare brought even more change. While it increased hospital business by making healthcare accessible to the elderly and poor, it also required independent auditors. Until this time, the church had audited its hospitals. While some resisted giving up this responsibility, like many other changes, this too came to pass.

Wages for healthcare employees was probably the most hotly contested issue. Traditionally, their pay was based on the church's ministerial wage scale, which was significantly less than other hospitals paid, making it extremely difficult to attract top-notch people. Clinical employees such as nurses, pharmacists, medical technologists and X-ray technologists were among the first to receive a community wage. Administrators would come later.

In Los Angeles County, tax-exempt hospitals had to submit a list of their top 50 wage earners each year. According to Dupper, who prepared these reports for Glendale, Remboldt's name never appeared on the list. As it became increasingly difficult to hire administrators at the ministerial wage, time came for change or risk losing the hospitals.

Another significant change came about during Remboldt's administration. A civic advisory board recommended removing the word "Sanitarium" from the name because it no longer reflected the hospital's business. When it was changed to Glendale Adventist Hospital on January 1, 1966, it was the first hospital in the United States to use "Adventist" in its name.

The 1960s brought other milestones, too. In 1966 Glendale Adventist was the first private hospital in Los Angeles to install the new 1440 IBM computer. A year later construction on the Ventura Freeway ate up 3.5 acres of hospital property. That same year ground was broken for a $3.5 million diagnostic and treatment center.

A Health System Begins

Remboldt was administrator of Glendale Adventist in 1972 when church leaders asked him to organize a corporation of Adventist hospitals in California, Arizona, Hawaii and Utah. He left the hospital in October 1973 to devote attention to the organization originally known as Adventist Health Services.

With large for-profit hospital corporations posing a real threat to the church's many stand-alone hospitals, discussions of uniting Adventist hospitals had been going on for some time. This would give them increased purchasing power, management expertise, economies of scale and marketing clout that they did not have on their own. Remboldt pioneered the system of Adventist hospitals in the western United States.

Before getting too involved in his new responsibilities, however, one of his first tasks was to set up an office for Adventist Health Services.

"We found a place down on Chevy Chase," he recalls. "I think it had four or five rooms. The secretary and I sat there the first day. We got two phone calls."

The calm did not last long because he soon began meeting with various hospital board members, trying to convince them to turn over their hospitals to this new organization—a job he describes as "no small feat." The first programs Adventist Health Services organized were malpractice insurance, purchasing and internal auditing.

Sometime later, Remboldt was also appointed president of Northwest Medical Foundation, which consisted of three hospitals in Washington and Oregon (Walla Walla General Hospital, Portland Adventist Hospital and Tillamook County General Hospital.) Adventist Health Services and Northwest Medical Foundation united in 1980 to form what is today's Adventist Health based in Roseville, California.

Time brought more changes to the Glendale hospital. A family practice residency program began in 1973. The main building of the 1923 hospital was replaced in the mid-1970s and the name was changed to Glendale Adventist Medical Center in 1975. Other milestones included the community's only neonatal intensive care unit opened in 1976, the MRI Institute in 1985, and the Physicians Medical Terrace in 1993. Today Glendale Adventist Medical Center is a 463-bed state-of-the-art medical facility.

SOURCES

Johns, Warren L., and Richard H. Utt, editors, *The Vision Bold*, Washington, D.C.: Review and Herald Publishing Association, 1977.

Judd, Wayne, tape recorded interviews with Don Ammon, Frank Dupper and Erwin Remboldt, 1998.

Interviews and Notes: Dr. Robert Horner, George Nelson and Erwin Remboldt.

Chapter 9

Not for Any Common Purpose

Loma Linda University Medical Center

Established 1905

An Educational Center

*"Loma Linda is not only a sanitarium, but an educational center.
With the possession of this place comes the weighty responsibility of
making the work of the institution educational in character. A school is to
be established here for the training of gospel medical missionary evangelists. Much is involved in this work, and it is very essential that a right
beginning be made. The Lord has a special work to be done in this part of
the field."* —ELLEN WHITE

When it appeared that the differences between church leaders and Dr.
John Harvey Kellogg could not be rectified, Ellen White began looking
for another location for a medical school. She urged church leaders to
explore some bargain properties in Southern California. Finally a committee headed by John Burden, business manager of the Glendale Sanitarium,
found a likely location near San Bernardino—a 76-acre resort called
Loma Linda with a hotel, farmhouse, cottages, amusement center and
other buildings. A group of businessmen and physicians had paid $15,000
for the property, and after investing another $155,000 in it, suffered a
downturn in business during the 1890s. Some even nicknamed the place
"Lonesome Linda."

When Burden found the property on the market for $110,000, he
knew it was far more than the church could afford—even if leaders
ignored their pay-as-you-go policy. With the recent establishment of the
Glendale Sanitarium, the church's Southern California Conference had no
money, and many church members who might have had the means to
invest had already put their money into the Paradise Valley project near
San Diego.

Even when the price dropped to $85,000, Burden could not consider
it. But when it came down to $40,000, he wrote to Mrs. White, who was in

Washington, D.C., at the time. She told him to "Secure the property by all means." She insisted, "This is the very property we ought to have."

Members of the local church conference were not so enthusiastic. With some committee members also in Washington, the rest did not feel at liberty to spend that kind of money without consulting their colleagues. They wired Washington and received a prompt-but-negative response.

What should Burden do? Mrs. White said go, and the brethren said no. More wires were exchanged between Washington and California until the order came, signed by Mrs. White, to do nothing until the church leaders returned to California. She later told Burden she could not ask the church to take on additional debt.

Burden knew that in her heart she did not want to wait. Mrs. White had once assured him the money would come from unexpected sources, and he believed with all his heart that it would. He tried to get an extension on the option to buy the property, but the owners insisted on $1,000 earnest money. Yet another message came from Washington: "Developments do not warrant securing Loma Linda." Fearing he would lose the sale, Burden signed the papers in his own name and bought the property.

When Mrs. White saw it, she was delighted with Loma Linda. "The Lord has not given us this property for any common purpose," she said.

Meanwhile, Burden had payments due, and his appeals to area churches seemed to generate more controversy than money. After the denomination's vice president G.A. Irwin began asking church members for assistance, gifts began coming—many from unexpected sources. One woman pledged $10,000. A letter from Atlantic City, New Jersey, contained $5,000. Another from Oregon contained $4,500. Within seven months the entire note was paid. With a discount for early payment, plus interest and taxes, Loma Linda was purchased for less than $46,000.

The new owners immediately began making repairs and renovations. Even though the Loma Linda Sanitarium did not officially open until November 1905, patients were coming in October. It was dedicated in April 1906, subsequently named Loma Linda College of Evangelists, and within only eight months, showed a gain of $1,160.

It took time to clarify the nature of the new college because some thought it was to train medical missionaries in simple treatments such as hydrotherapy and massage while others believed it must be an accredited school for training fully qualified physicians. Ellen White's comment that the school was to be "of the highest order," gave leaders a clear directive.

The name was changed to College of Medical Evangelists and the newly appointed leaders included Dr. Wells Allen Ruble, president, Dr. George K. Abbott, dean, John Burden, business manager, and G.A. Irwin, board chairman. The first faculty members were mostly former teachers and graduates of American Medical Missionary College in Battle Creek.

Until the early 1900s, almost anyone could start a medical school in the United States, and these institutions were cranking out diplomas almost as fast as they could print them. Some did not even require a high school diploma for admission. The best schools offered only 24 months of training.

In an effort to close some of these schools and upgrade the professional training for physicians, the American Medical Association set up a rating system. Most states allowed only graduates of A and B schools to take their board examinations, leaving a degree from a C-rated school virtually worthless.

Although representatives of the rating organization advised closing the College of Medical Evangelists in 1912, school leaders would not think of it. They continued with limited resources but great faith. One of the big problems was finding sufficient clinical experience for the students in Loma Linda. As a solution, the school set up a program with the Los Angeles County Hospital, and also opened a dispensary in Los Angeles. In spite of these efforts, CME received a C rating in 1914.

Some considered this proof enough that the church should exit the medical school business. Others suggested cutting back to a two-year curriculum. Finally the clinical program in Los Angeles was strengthened and the four-year program continued. When the decision was made in 1915 to build a $60,000 hospital in Los Angeles, President Evans recommended Dr. Percy Magan, his former associate at Madison College in Tennessee, be invited to develop the Los Angeles campus. Magan accepted the position of dean, and led the school through challenges that he said were "beset with difficulties from every side."

Long Road to Loma Linda

Magan was the kind of person who made a big difference in whatever he did. Born in Ireland in 1867, he moved to the United States in his teens, and became a Seventh-day Adventist. He soon attracted the attention of Nellie Druillard, a teacher and church official in Nebraska, who encouraged him to attend Battle Creek College. There he met Druillard's nephew, Edward Sutherland, who became his lifelong friend, colleague and confidant.

At Mrs. White's recommendation Magan accompanied evangelist Stephen Haskell on a historic round-the-world mission tour in 1890. The trip, chronicled in a series of 49 articles in "The Youth's Instructor" during 1890 and 1891, made a profound impression on the young man and helped form his philosophy of education.

With his friend Sutherland, Magan had built the Madison school from the ground up, and it was not easy to leave in 1915. However, he knew the future of Madison—as well as other Adventist hospitals—depended on having qualified physicians. Developing CME into an A-level school was a huge challenge as he dealt with faculty and organizational issues, accreditation, fundraising, and attitudes ranging from indifference to outright opposition.

He kept his friend Sutherland abreast of the challenges. When he told him he needed $60,000 to build White Memorial Hospital, Sutherland arranged to send $50,000 from Madison. (See Chapter 12 on Tennessee Christian Medical Center.)

The medical school board authorized the purchase of a half block of property in the Boyle Heights area of Los Angeles. Knowing it was far too small, Magan told Evans one day that he would not show his Irish face again until he had the money to buy the rest of the block. While the board later reprimanded him for buying the land without authorization, he felt that was a small price to pay for the future of the school.

Before the property had been developed, Magan took Dr. Nathan P. Colwell to see it. Colwell had been a member of the committee that advised Adventists to give up the school in 1912. As the two men looked at the "mass of weeds, cockleburs, and...two or three sorry-looking animals" feeding on the property, Magan told him that one day a great medical organization would occupy the site.

"You poor soul," Colwell thought. "You do not know what you are talking about,"

In time, of course, Magan would prove him wrong.

During World War I the C-rated school was at risk of losing some faculty and students to the draft, which could jeopardize its future. Magan knew if the school closed it would never reopen. He personally visited the Surgeon General in Washington, D.C., and the medical school rating agency in Chicago. It took some creative negotiating and answers to prayer, but in the end CME received an early inspection and the B classification it needed for students and faculty to be deferred from the draft.

The school faced another crisis in 1921 when an accrediting committee found it to be weak in several key areas, specifically the divided campus, insufficient budget and lack of research facilities. It took much persuasion and many prayers, but the changes were made, and the medical school finally received an A classification in 1922. No one was more surprised than Colwell.

"I feel ashamed of myself sitting here rating you people...while you are doing the really big things of the world," he told Magan. "You have done wonders in your school...."

After serving as dean from 1915 to 1928, Magan was president of CME until 1942.

♈

The 1960s saw major changes for the school, which was renamed Loma Linda University in 1961. Under Dr. David Hinshaw's direction, the two-campus arrangement ended by relocating the clinical programs to Loma Linda—a highly controversial issue that sharply divided the faculty as well as church leaders and members. (See Chapter 15 on White Memorial Medical Center.)

All-day Debate

I was present at the Annual Council in 1962 when the decision was made to consolidate the medical school at Loma Linda. The discussion took a whole day. There was a parade of speakers, some urging Loma Linda and others Los Angeles. The great fear was that there wouldn't be enough clinical opportunities in the Loma Linda area. I attended 25 Annual Councils in future years, but I can't remember another more hotly debated issue. When the vote was finally taken late that night, it was for Loma Linda by a strong majority. —WILLIAM MURRILL, RETIRED UNDERTREASURER, GENERAL CONFERENCE OF SEVENTH-DAY ADVENTISTS

♈

The opening of the $20 million Loma Linda University Medical Center in 1967 marked a new era for the organization. In the book *Legacy*, author Richard A. Schaefer reports that within the next 30 years the hospital grew 600 percent. Today it is a multi-campus medical center, teaching facility and research center, with internationally recognized programs in organ transplantation, cancer treatment, rehabilitation, orthopaedics, perinatal biology and cardiac surgery. The Loma Linda University Heart Surgery Team has performed more heart surgeries in more countries than any other similar organization.

It was a special heart surgery that gained Loma Linda University Medical Center international attention in 1984. At that time the name Baby Fae was permanently etched in the history pages of medical science when she underwent transplantation of a baboon's heart. While the procedure drew both approval and condemnation, it was a landmark case.

"It has become a reference point in the public's awareness of hypoplastic left-heart syndrome and the serious efforts being made to save doomed babies," writes Schaffer. "It became the cornerstone of a successful, international, infant-to-infant heart-transplant program begun in Loma Linda about a year later."

Hope for Special Babies

This story begins shortly after the first successful human-heart transplant in 1967 by Dr. Christiaan Barnard in South Africa. Leonard Bailey, a medical student at Loma Linda, began studying heart transplantation in 1969. After medical school, he took a residency at the Hospital for Sick Children in Toronto, Canada, where he specialized in pediatric cardiac surgery. He was especially interested in hypoplastic left-heart syndrome, the underdevelopment of the left side of the heart, which occurs about once in every 12,000 live births in the United States.

At Loma Linda, Dr. Bailey and his associates were seeing from six to eight babies die every year as a result of hypoplastic left-heart syndrome, and began to look at transplantation as a solution. After six years of research and many months of working through the approval process, the door was finally opened for a cross-species transplant at Loma Linda.

A baby girl with hypoplastic left-heart syndrome was born prematurely in Barstow, California, in October 1984. The mother discussed the procedure at length with Bailey, and while he could give her no guarantee of success, she knew her baby had no other chance at life.

Many sophisticated and time-consuming tests were done to find the best tissue-matched donor, during which time Baby Fae almost died. Meanwhile, the hospital's institutional review board monitored the situation closely, granting its final approval only two days before the surgery.

The baby's condition had stabilized by the time the test results were received at 4 a.m., Friday, October 26. The history-making surgery began at 6:30 a.m., taking doctors about one hour to implant the walnut-size heart in the baby's chest. By 11:35 a.m., it was beating on its own.

Although Baby Fae lived only 20 days, she and her family made an immeasurable contribution in the effort to save babies born with a lethal abnormality.

Loma Linda University Medical Center made a major commitment to treating cancer and other diseases with the opening of the first hospital-based proton-beam accelerator in 1990. The $85 million, three-story facility represents a major advancement in treating localized tumors because the proton beam can target them without damaging surrounding tissue. In 2001 Loma Linda was treating about 140 patients every day with this type of cancer therapy.

Other scientific contributions of note by Loma Linda include the development of pallidotomy surgery for sufferers of Parkinson's disease, and the use of human-computer interface technology to help people with severe physical handicaps.

Except for the hill on which it was built, today's Loma Linda University bears no resemblance to the "Lonesome Linda" health resort of the early 1900s. Tens of thousands have graduated from the university's schools of medicine, dentistry, public health, nursing and allied health. Clearly, Loma Linda University and the Loma Linda University Medical Center bear witness to the statement made nearly a century ago that God did not provide this place for any common purpose.

SOURCES

Gish, Ira, and Harry Christman, *Madison—God's Beautiful Farm*, Nampa, Idaho: The Upward Way, 1989.

Johns, Warren L., and Richard H. Utt, editors, *The Vision Bold*, Washington, D.C.: Review and Herald Publishing Association, 1977.

Neff, Merlin L., *For God and C.M.E.*, Mountain View, California: Pacific Press Publishing Association, 1964.

Schaefer, Richard A., *Legacy: Daring to Care,* Loma Linda, California: Legacy Publishing Association, 1995.

Utt, Richard, *From Vision to Reality*, Loma Linda, California: Loma Linda University, 1980.

Interview and Notes: William Murrill.

Chapter 10

When David Paulson Prayed

Hinsdale Hospital
Established 1905

$5,000 Answer to Prayer

Shortly before Hinsdale Sanitarium opened, Dr. David Paulson needed to pay some bills, and borrowed $5,000 from a wealthy Hinsdale resident named Dr. Pearsons. He later needed another $5,000 and Pearsons loaned the funds again—on the condition that the whole $10,000 would be repaid by April 1.

Two weeks before the deadline, Pearsons asked the doctor whether he had the money. Paulson said no, but assured him he would have it by April 1.

"Where can you get it?" Pearsons asked.

Paulson said he would look to the Lord for it.

Two days before the deadline, a sanitarium visitor approached the doctor after morning worship. She said she was expecting to receive $5,000 and thought perhaps he could use it. A few hours later Pearsons showed up at the business office, announcing that he had persuaded a local bank to loan the sanitarium $5,000. With the money the woman had promised, Paulson had all he needed to pay the bills.

Adventist healthcare in Chicago was a product of Dr. John Harvey Kellogg's work in Battle Creek. It started in 1892 when a wealthy man put up the money for a nurse to work among Chicago's poor.

Sometime later John Wessels, a Seventh-day Adventist whose family had made a fortune in the diamond mines of South Africa, asked Kellogg what he would do if he were to receive a large amount of money. When Kellogg said he would open a mission for the poor in Chicago, Wessels gave him $40,000.

At that time, the young man who would eventually direct this mission work and establish Hinsdale Hospital was studying at the University of Michigan. However, David Paulson's story began several years earlier during an outbreak of diphtheria in South Dakota. In the book *His Name was David*, Paulson's sister-in-law, Caroline Louise Clough, describes how the illness devastated the Paulson family.

A Promise for Life

"Martin is dead. You must help me carry him out," David heard his father tell one of his brothers.

When they returned to the house, the sick boy heard his father's voice again.

"David will be next. He can't last long. I think we had better wait and bury both boys at once."

As he lay in bed, David promised that if he were allowed to live, he would devote his life to helping the sick and suffering—a promise he faithfully kept throughout his lifetime.

Paulson attended Battle Creek College and in 1891 was one of several students selected to study medicine at the University of Michigan. From Ann Arbor, he moved to New York City to complete his studies at Bellevue Medical College. He worked in the medical mission operated by Dr. George Dowkontt in the slums of New York, and during this time he visited many homes where people had little food and few comforts of life. It made a lasting impression on him.

Although Dowkontt dreamed of starting a medical school in New York, one morning it occurred to Paulson that the school should be established in Michigan. He did not know that Kellogg had already begun plans for a medical school at Battle Creek.

When he left New York, Paulson joined the mission work in Chicago, which grew rapidly with clinics, dispensaries, a branch sanitarium, a home for unwed mothers and their babies, a men's mission, a magazine and much more. It soon was large enough to provide the clinical practice for medical students at the new American Medical Missionary College, which opened in 1895 with campuses in Battle Creek and Chicago.

Stenographer's Prayer

One day Paulson prayed for a stenographer to assist in recording his lectures. Only a couple of days later, a man in ragged clothes came asking for work. At first the doctor was sure he had no job for the unkempt man.

"I'm a stenographer, sir," the man said.

Without hesitating, the two men knelt and thanked God for bringing them together. This man turned out to be an outstanding stenographer, who could recall Paulson's lectures almost verbatim without taking notes.

Another day Paulson and a patient named C.B. Kimbell were talking about the mission's work for unwed mothers. The facility being used for these women was in an area with many saloons and brothels, and most of the mothers returned to the very lifestyle that had brought them to the mission in the first place. Paulson needed a facility away from the city for the women and their babies. Kimbell offered him a house in Hinsdale, which met the need nicely.

The Chicago mission work lost its financial support after the Battle Creek Sanitarium burned in 1902, and it was clear that Adventist healthcare in that city must take another direction. Expressing concern that the mission work was a financial drain on the denomination, Ellen White called for a balance that would provide for the needy while attracting a clientele that could pay for services.

Paulson was firmly committed to the poor and feared losing this aspect of the church's mission if it built a sanitarium that catered to the wealthy. At one point he made an impassioned plea to board members, saying he was "determined there shall be one spot left on this selfish earth where a man can have a helping hand extended to him whether he has money or not." Once again, his friend Kimbell came up with a solution: Build a sanitarium first for those who can pay, then establish a work for the sick poor.

Sometime later Kimbell took Paulson and his physician wife, Mary, to a property that might be suitable for a sanitarium. It was the Judge Beckwith home, a 10-acre wooded estate in Hinsdale with a 15-room house, plus another nine-room structure and plenty of outbuildings. The $16,000 price tag certainly was right, but the Paulsons had not one cent to buy it. A few days later Kimbell came back with an offer.

"I'll buy the property and deed it to you on the basis that you pay for it in 20 yearly installments without interest," he said.

Rooftop Prayers

Plans for the sanitarium continued with many answered prayers. Shortly before opening the new facility, Paulson needed $1,000 to complete the roof. Once again he called the sanitarium family together to pray and a few days later he received a letter with a check.

"I hear you are trying to start a sanitarium in Hinsdale," the writer said. "I have just sold my farm and have $1,150 to place somewhere. I don't know why, but I feel urged to send it to you."

The sanitarium opened in 1905, with the first inpatient arriving before the stairs were completed. Thanks to a dumb waiter not yet removed from the building, the staff lifted the patient to the upper floor.

By 1910 the College of Medical Evangelists had started in California and American Medical Missionary College—with all the clinics and dispensaries connected with the Chicago Medical Mission—had closed. In that same year Paulson realized his dream of a facility on the sanitarium campus for the sick poor.

Good Samaritan Prayer

"About the time we were making our last enlargement of the sanitarium and building the Rescue Home, we felt the time had come to definitely establish our work for the sick poor, the Good Samaritan Inn...but strangely enough I could not get hold of any money to put in a heating plant...the house was cold and the patients had to be moved over to the sanitarium...It actually took us a couple of years more before we were again able to open our Good Samaritan Inn...When we did, a good woman gave us four hundred dollars without any solicitation, to make the necessary repairs....

"One night a stranger who happened to be here, sent for me after I had gone home and wanted me to tell him about the Good Samaritan Inn, which I did. He wrote me a check for one hundred dollars. Next one of our patients, without my having mentioned the matter to her, sent me one hundred dollars for the same purpose, and another good woman gave me a hundred dollars." —DR. DAVID PAULSON

Paulson became gravely ill in 1916. After short stays at Madison, Tennessee, and Boulder, Colorado, the 48-year-old doctor moved near Asheville, North Carolina. However, his health was spent, and his condition gradually worsened. Two noteworthy visitors came to his bedside before he died, Dr. Percy Magan from Tennessee, and cereal giant W.K. Kellogg, who paid for his funeral expenses and transportation back to Hinsdale.

Over the years, Hinsdale Sanitarium had its ups and downs, but it was always successful and highly regarded. One of the most noted chapters in its history occurred during a polio epidemic in 1949. In one month alone

13 cases were reported in the community, and the number approached 70 before the epidemic ended. People hated to hear their phones ring for fear it would be news of another polio case.

Eugene Kettering, son of inventor Charles F. Kettering, and his family had recently moved near the sanitarium, when the son of one of their landscape workers was diagnosed with polio. Because the sanitarium was not equipped for this type of care, he was taken to another hospital. A short time later, the Ketterings equipped a unit for contagious diseases at the sanitarium.

"Everyone wanted to do something," Virginia Kettering said.

Christmas Gift for Polio Patients

In the early days of the polio epidemic, the hospital had no iron lungs. The story is told that Mrs. Kettering asked her daughter what she wanted for Christmas.

"Mother, you know I don't need anything," the young girl said.

"Yes, you do," Mrs. Kettering replied. "You need three new iron lungs for the Hinsdale San to treat the polio patients."

Eugene Kettering personally arranged for the iron lungs to be transported and delivered to the Hinsdale San. —RAY PELTON, RETIRED ASSOCIATE DIRECTOR, HEALTH AND TEMPERANCE DEPARTMENT, GENERAL CONFERENCE OF SEVENTH-DAY ADVENTISTS

The Ketterings went to the hospital every night, taking food the community had prepared for the staff. Describing the therapists as "the most beautiful people," Mrs. Kettering said she believed their care and attention made all the difference in the patients' progress.

By the end of the year the Ketterings had organized a major fund-raising effort to replace the old wooden structure in which the Paulsons had started the Hinsdale Sanitarium 50 years earlier. The new hospital opened in 1953.

Early Lessons in Hospital Management

Hinsdale Hospital has been the starting place for a number of Adventist healthcare leaders, among them Ray Pelton, who later was administrator of White Memorial Medical Center and New England Memorial Hospital, as well as an associate at the church's world headquarters.

With a brand new degree from Union College in Lincoln, Nebraska, young Pelton arrived at Hinsdale in 1949 expecting an entry-level

position with some management responsibility. Instead, he was an orderly. It seems that the person in the position for which Pelton had been hired was in no hurry to move. After two or three months as an orderly Pelton was promoted to night admitting clerk—a job that taught him some valuable lessons in working with the public.

One night a man dressed in a lumberman's flannel shirt came into the hospital with a young woman who was being admitted. He identified himself as Mr. Evans.

"And what is your daughter's name?" Pelton asked.

"This is my wife," Evans said, correcting him.

The embarrassed Pelton would later learn that the gentleman with the young wife was the owner of Chicago's famous Evans Hotel and the builder of the elevated train track in the Chicago Loop.

A.C. Larson was administrator of Hinsdale Sanitarium and Hospital from 1954 to 1963. Although he was regarded as a kind gentleman, he didn't stand for any foolishness. Pelton admits to having been corrected on occasion by the no-nonsense leader.

"He was democratic, but he called the shots," says Pelton, recalling the experience of one employee that Larson had determined needed to find another career opportunity. This man boasted that he had no intention of leaving his position. "Administrators come and go, but I stay," he said.

A few weeks later the employee did not receive a paycheck. Needless to say, he left Hinsdale and Larson stayed.

Larson was the first of nine Hinsdale administrators with whom Kathryn Sieberman, retired vice president, worked between 1957 and 1999. Each had his unique style and contributed to the hospital's success.

"Even though it seemed he was strictly all business, Mr. Larson had a very kind heart. He did things to help employees feel like family—picnics, corn roasts, watermelon feeds, Christmas parties and Saturday night lyceums," says Sieberman.

Among her favorite memories of the Larson era were the visits of his brother-in-law, Harley Rice.

"He was 'Mr. Hospital' in the Adventist church in those days and traveled around the world helping medical institutions," she recalls. "He was also a poet and wrote about his travels. When he visited Hinsdale, Mr. Larson would invite him to have morning worship for the administrative staff, which met every morning promptly at eight o'clock in his office. Harley Rice would give us wonderful travelogues describing his visits to such places as Calcutta and Bangalore."

During the 1960s Sieberman worked with Mardian Blair and Bill Wilson, both administrators who devoted a lot of effort to recruiting a strong team of employees.

"One of us might go to Madison, Wisconsin, another to Indianapolis, and another to Detroit. We'd stay for three to five days, calling every church elder within any reasonable distance to get names of members who might be potential employees—nurses, nurse's aides, cooks, accountants, secretaries. We'd come home from those trips with about 30 names," she explains. "Then we'd have to sort them out."

Hinsdale's Great Dane

Anyone who has been around Hinsdale Hospital for any time has likely heard of Anna Viola Pedersen, affectionately known as "Anna Pete." She went to Hinsdale when she was only 19 years old and worked at the hospital for 57 years. She loved to tell people, "I'm a Great Dane. I was born in Copenhagen!"

Whatever she did, Anna Pete did it well, whether it was housekeeping, food service, laundry or elevator operator. A good cook, she often prepared midnight supper for the night staff, who especially liked her potato soup made with cream.

Anna Pete never married and had few relatives. She lived in a one-room apartment owned by the hospital. There she grew amaryllis plants, which she never kept for herself. Even in her advanced years, when she walked with a cane, she personally delivered her amaryllis blooms to the hospital information desk for others to enjoy.

When she retired, well in her 80s, she feared having to move from the apartment, but the hospital allowed her to stay. Today the building in which she lived is called Anna Pedersen Hall in her honor.

I saw that Anna Pete had her medicines and took care of her until she could no longer walk. At that point she was moved to a private home where she died in 1972 at age 94. Anna Pete is buried in a hospital cemetery lot with 24 other former employees—only steps away from the graves of David and Mary Paulson, founders of the hospital where this Great Dane served for more than half a century. —KATHRYN SIEBERMAN

SOURCES

Clough, Caroline Louise, *His Name was David*, Washington, D.C.: Review and Herald Publishing Association, 1955.

Dugan, Hugh G., *Hinsdale Sanitarium and Hospital 1904 to 1957*. (Publisher and date unknown.)

"Hinsdale Hospital: Weaving a Tapestry Through Ninety Years of Caring," *Visions*, Anniversary Issue, 1995.

Nelson, George, *The Kettering Medical Center: Recollections and Reflections of the Early Years, 1996.*

Paulson, David, *Footprints of Faith*, Hinsdale, Illinois: Life Boat Publishing Company, 1921.

Robinson, D.E., *The Story of Our Health Message*, Nashville, Tennessee: Southern Publishing Association, 1965.

Interviews: Ray Pelton and Katherine Sieberman.

Chapter 11

Healthy Spot on God's Footstool

Washington Adventist Hospital
Established 1907

Designed by Nature

Sometime in the 1880s two community leaders walked over the undeveloped land above Sligo Creek in Takoma Park, Maryland. They noticed the sound of water below could be heard more clearly from one particular spot than from any other point. One commented that "nature had designed this place" for a healthcare facility. Later a physician named Dr. Flower cleared part of the 50-acre site to build a medical institution, but after investing about $60,000 in the project, he never finished it.

Several years later leaders of the Seventh-day Adventist Church found this property not far from the Washington, D.C., line and bought it for only $6,000.

ॐ

While today's Columbia Union College was established on this property in 1904, it would take three more years to open a sanitarium in Takoma Park. In the meantime, Adventists rented the former residence of Ulysses S. Grant on Iowa Circle (now Logan Circle) in Washington, D.C. In this large house they opened a "Branch San," which operated from 1904 until 1914. Patrons included many government officials and their families.

Meanwhile, in Takoma Park construction of a four-story structure with large verandas began in 1906. The following year the Washington Sanitarium and a school of nursing opened with Drs. Daniel and Lauretta Kress as the first medical director and surgeon, respectively. In fact, Dr. Lauretta was the first licensed woman physician in Montgomery County. Dr. Daniel would serve as medical director from 1907 to 1909 and again from 1937 to 1938.

The Kresses had studied and worked at Battle Creek in the late 1800s, and between 1899 and 1907 helped establish healthcare facilities in Great Britain, Australia and New Zealand. In many ways the Washington

Sanitarium was another mission field. As Dr. Daniel explains in the autobiography he co-authored with his wife, the San was in the country and accessible only by undeveloped roads. Although built to accommodate 35 patients, few people knew about the San and often the staff outnumbered patients.

An Early Plea for Equal Pay

The Kresses devoted themselves to making the Washington Sanitarium succeed—a point that Dr. Daniel made clear to officials when he asked that Dr. Lauretta be paid the same salary as he did. He explained that she spent as much or more time on her job as he, and received only $15 a week, compared to his $20.

"Rent is high, and we have to keep a woman employed as Mrs. Kress gives no attention whatever to her home duties. Her time is given entirely to the San," he wrote in a letter to officials.

Apparently she received the raise. In the autobiography, she reports receiving $20 a week plus a "Ford runabout car" that had no self-starter and had to be cranked.

Though Dr. Lauretta's primary responsibility was chief surgeon, she also headed the maternity department. During her 31 years at the Washington Sanitarium, she delivered more than 5,000 babies.

In the early days the Washington Sanitarium may have been one of the best-kept secrets in the area, but those who patronized it spoke highly of the location and the care they received. Among those guests was the superintendent of government gardens, who wrote an article for the *Washington Star* newspaper applauding the facility and calling it "the healthiest spot on God's footstool."

Rural Attraction

"Seekers of the picturesque will be delighted with the scenes which present themselves in quick succession, along one of the most delightful rural drives through the healthiest region around Washington, in fact, not surpassed anywhere...God's great out-of-doors, combined with the rational treatments, the hygienic diet, and the spiritual atmosphere which pervades the institution, make this an ideal place for health seekers or for those who feel the need of an occasional period of rest and recreation."

Life at the early Washington Sanitarium was also typical of Adventist health centers of that time. Guests attended lectures, ate in the dining room and worked in the sanitarium gardens. For recreation they exercised in the gymnasium and played croquet, shuffleboard and golf. A sanitarium orchestra also frequently provided entertainment.

In order for the Washington Sanitarium to succeed, two important things were needed—patients and money. When Dr. Harry Miller, the famous missionary physician in China, returned to the United States in 1911 due to illness, church leaders asked him to head the Washington San. After he had recovered sufficiently, in 1913 he assumed the dual position as medical director of the sanitarium and director of the denomination's worldwide medical work. He was acquainted with the Drs. Kress. In fact, many years earlier, Dr. Daniel had encouraged him to study medicine at Battle Creek.

The San was still paying off its building debt in 1913. Also, there had been a typhoid epidemic among the employees, resulting in a low patient census. Miller said patient rounds during his early days there consisted primarily of shaking hands with three or four old women. In fact, to keep active in surgery, he reportedly opened an animal hospital on the back lawn of the sanitarium.

The financial situation began to improve after word spread that Miller had successfully performed a very difficult surgery. He also took post-graduate work in thyroid surgery and soon the San became a thriving thyroid center. The doctor donated his fees to the sanitarium, saving only enough to meet his personal expenses.

Business outgrew the original facility by 1916, and Miller recommended constructing a separate building for surgery. With the memory of high debt still in their minds, the board said no. Miller went ahead anyway, and by the time the board members learned of it, the roofers were already at work. Even though Miller promised the building would be paid for within a year, it actually opened debt-free—paid for mostly from his thyroid-surgery fees.

Patients were coming to the Washington Sanitarium from near and far, representing many walks of life—from government officials and foreign diplomats to charity patients—and sometimes with unexpected results. For example, one patient told his family and friends about his experience at the Washington Sanitarium, and as a result, Drs. Miller and Kress were asked to help establish a sanitarium in Greeneville, Tennessee. (See Chapter 17 on Takoma Adventist Hospital.)

Miller remained in Takoma Park until he returned to China in 1925. The Kresses stayed until 1938. Dr. Daniel specialized in narcotics education and made a significant contribution to the field before he and Dr. Lauretta retired in Florida.

Of the Washington Sanitarium Dr. Daniel once commented that it must have been "a source of the greatest satisfaction" for the founder of Takoma Park to know that the land he had judged to be ideal for a sanitarium had indeed proven to be so. Kress believed that the San had reached its potential by 1932 when he made the following statement at the facility's 25th anniversary.

It's Big Enough

"The institution has now reached its full growth, since there exists no expectation of enlarging it any further. We believe it to be sufficiently large to do its best work." —DR. DANIEL KRESS

Time brought many changes the Kresses could never have imagined as the sanitarium grew into a modern acute-care hospital. The main entrance was moved in 1939 from the side facing Sligo Creek to the side facing the college. A six-story structure built in 1950 replaced the old buildings that had made up the main part of the hospital, leaving many to wonder how the San would ever pay for the "extravagant" $1.4 million facility.

Among other developments, the 1960s saw the addition of an intensive-care unit, school of X-ray technology, school of practical nursing, alcohol treatment center and coronary-care unit. Also during this time Chaplain Alfred Marple brought to Washington the Five-Day Plan to Stop Smoking. During his 35 years at the hospital, he personally helped more than 50,000 people complete the stop-smoking program. In addition to offering classes at the hospital, he took the plan to various government offices in Washington, D.C.

The sanitarium's name was changed to Washington Adventist Hospital in the early 1970s, and a $12.5 million expansion increased the patient bed capacity to 366. Although the hospital later reduced the number of patient beds to 300, construction and growth continued throughout the 1990s.

While some worried about the increasing cost of hospital expansion, it was a demolition project that created a loud outcry from the local community and church members. The original 1907 sanitarium building—a stately old structure that had been a landmark in Takoma Park for most of a century—did not meet fire and safety codes and was condemned for patient use. Additionally, the cost of heating and cooling the structure was excessive, as was the cost of maintaining the old wood and stucco building. Hospital leaders figured it would take $1.2 million to renovate the building, a cost that would have to be passed on to patients. Even with renovations, the facility would be inadequate. So, amid voices of protest, the building was demolished in 1982.

Today Washington Adventist Hospital is the oldest operating hospital in Montgomery County, Maryland. While the peaceful, rural setting of the original facility has given way to modern urbanization, the hospital continues the mission on which it was established nearly a century ago, meeting the physical, mental and spiritual needs of those who come for care.

SOURCES

Jepson, Robert E., "A.C. Marple Kicks the Habit," *Visitor*, September 1, 1995.

Kress, Daniel and Lauretta, *Under the Guiding Hand*, Washington, D.C.: College Press, 1941.

Moore, Raymond S., *China Doctor,* Mt. View, California: Pacific Press Publishing Association, 1969.

"90 Years of Progress Spring from a Mission of Caring," 1979.

Interview and Notes: William Murrill.

Chapter 12

Rocky Venture on the Cumberland

Tennessee Christian Medical Center
Established 1908

Not What They Had in Mind

*"It's the roughest, weediest, most miserable thing I've ever seen,"
Edward Sutherland told Percy Magan as they looked around the
rock-covered Ferguson-Nelson farm near Nashville, Tennessee.*

*Ellen White said this was the land where God wanted them to start a
training school. They argued that it was run down, and much too big and
expensive for their budget. But it was hard to argue with Mrs. White, who
said they were making their plans too small and setting their aim too low.*

*"If you will follow the counsel of the Lord, He will set your feet in a
large place and provide the money to pay for it," she said.*

*Now, sitting on one of the many rocks that populated the barren farm,
Sutherland and Magan cried.*

*"It does me up and makes me sick, the whole thought of it," Suther-
land said. "I wish we had some honorable and Christian way to get out of
the whole thing without showing lack of faith in the testimonies from the
Lord's messenger."*

The two men knelt and prayed, and then went home.

*The next day they returned, and again they sat on the rock, and again
they prayed, begging God to show His will. This time their fears subsided,
and God's answer seemed crystal clear. They must buy the property.*

The earliest Adventist medical work around Nashville began in the
late 1890s with small treatment rooms offering massage and
hydrotherapy, but these were never financially successful. In fact, the
church's medical work did not get a solid footing here until after a
self-supporting school and sanitarium were established in Madison, home
of today's Tennessee Christian Medical Center. Ellen White played a key
role at Madison from the very beginning, serving on the Nashville
Agricultural and Normal Institute (doing business as Madison Sanitarium

and Hospital and Madison College) board of directors until 1914, about a year before her death.

Magan and Sutherland, who had helped move Battle Creek College and establish Emmanuel Missionary College (today's Andrews University in Michigan), moved to Tennessee in 1904 to set up a new kind of school. They envisioned a place in the hills of Tennessee or the Carolinas where students would learn practical trades and simple medical treatments. They planned to begin small and let their work grow as they had money to expand. However, when they arrived in Nashville, Mrs. White was already there, and that changed everything.

Her son Edson White was operating a boat called *Morning Star*, traveling the rivers of the South to work among the African-American population. Like Magan and Sutherland, he was interested in starting a school. At Mrs. White's invitation Magan and Sutherland joined a small group on a trip up the Cumberland River to look for suitable property. Only a few miles from Nashville the boat broke down near an old plantation farm. While waiting for repairs, Mrs. White went ashore and walked around the rock-covered run down property that had once been a slave-trading center. She insisted this was the place Magan and Sutherland should establish their school.

A Visit to Aunt Nellie

While Magan remained in Nashville to work out the purchase, Sutherland went to Michigan to see his Aunt Nellie Druillard, hoping she would help them buy the Tennessee farm. A woman of unusual business skill, Druillard was treasurer of Emmanuel Missionary College at that time. Many years earlier, she and her husband had purchased property in Wyoming. Oil was discovered on the land after her husband's death, and she sold it for a large amount of money. Over the years she used her wealth to assist the church's health and education work.

When Sutherland told her about the farm, she thought it sounded like a "rocky" venture, to say the least. By this time, however, he was so convinced that the Lord had led in the selection of the property that he told her he would find money elsewhere if she would not help. At last she agreed to go to Nashville to look over the situation.

Mrs. White was in Madison again when Sutherland returned with his aunt. They soon learned of the troubles Magan had encountered with the property owner's wife, who at one point, declared she would never sell to a Yankee. Although she finally agreed to sell, she raised the price by $1,000. Authors Ira Gish and Harry Christman give the following account of the exchange between Druillard and Mrs. White when they heard this development.

It's Cheap Enough

"Ha," Mrs. Druillard exclaimed. "I'm glad we're not going to take it."

"Glad!" Mrs. White's voice rang out. "Glad! Do you think I'd let the devil beat me out of a place for a thousand dollars? Pay the extra thousand. It's cheap enough. This is the place the Lord said you should have."

In the end, Druillard was among those who joined the Madison school as a permanent staff member. She remained there for the rest of her life, except for eight years when she established Riverside Sanitarium (See Chapter 16).

First Patient Arrives

Soon after the opening of Nashville Agricultural and Normal Institute (later Madison College), a sick man came to the school. He told the staff that he believed he would recover if given proper rest, a healthy diet and the treatments they could give him. Although the school was not set up for patients, he insisted on staying.

Druillard hung a curtain on one end of a porch on the plantation house to make room for him, and she and three nursing students cared for him until he recovered. Afterward he told others about his experience, and demand for medical care at Madison began to grow.

The plan had always been to operate a sanitarium with the school, but there was hardly enough money available for school needs, let alone medical work. Besides, neither Sutherland nor Magan had any experience in running medical institutions. Again, Mrs. White had other ideas.

On a visit to Madison in 1906 she joined some students and faculty for a picnic. Enjoying the pleasant afternoon, she looked across the campus and announced, "This would be a good spot for a sanitarium." The response of the other picnickers was less than enthusiastic, but Mrs. White meant what she said.

"Get your people together and get a horse and mark out the site, even though you don't have money to begin," she said.

After lunch and a brief prayer meeting, someone hitched a mule to a plow and marked out the spot as she had told them to do.

The first medical building at Madison was a small cottage with 11 beds and treatment rooms. In *Madison—God's Beautiful Farm*, the authors describe a humble pioneer cottage lighted by kerosene lamps and equipped with a wood stove and treatment table made of a wide board on two wooden sawhorses.

The new Madison Rural Sanitarium desperately needed doctors. Magan's wife, Lillian, was the first staff physician. Dr. Newton Evans assisted her for a time, but then moved to the new Adventist medical school in California. Finally at the ages of 46 and 42 respectively, Sutherland and Magan enrolled in the University of Tennessee Medical School in Nashville. Local residents often saw them riding their motorcycles to and from school. They graduated in 1914, planning to strengthen the medical program at Madison, but 1915 brought an unexpected turn of events.

Magan was invited by his friend Evans to develop a clinical program for the struggling College of Medical Evangelists (CME) in California. It was a difficult separation for Magan and Sutherland, for they had worked together for many years and Madison was a fulfillment of their dreams. After Magan became dean at CME, other staff joined him in California, but Sutherland remained at Madison the rest of his life. Though separated by miles, the two men remained close friends and confidants.

Madison Helps the Medical School

When Magan saw that the medical school needed to build a hospital in Los Angeles, he turned to Sutherland, and his friend came through for him. Sutherland called on two women from the Madison area—Hetty Haskell, Bible instructor, teacher and wife of evangelist Stephen Haskell, and Josephine Gotzian, a woman of means who had generously assisted Madison, as well as other schools and hospitals. He told them to go to California and get together with Haskell's widowed sister, Emma Gray, and Dr. Florence Keller, teacher at the College of Medical Evangelists. (See Chapter 15 on White Memorial Medical Center.)

"Please go in the name and power of God and do what you can to save the medical school," Sutherland said.

It so happened that at this time a generous donor had promised a substantial gift to Madison for much-needed improvements. However, after hearing of the need in California, she agreed to send $30,000 to Magan. Eventually the Madison group increased the amount to $50,000.

Finances were always an issue for Madison because, as a self-supporting organization, it received little denominational assistance. To complicate matters, Madison leaders were notified in 1911 that they could no longer publish fund-raising articles or report their school and sanitarium activities in the church paper, *The Review and Herald*. Fortunately, Madison attracted the attention of three wealthy widows, including Druillard mentioned above.

Generous Women of Means

Josephine Gotzian and her husband, a shoe manufacturer, had been in a train accident in which he was killed and she suffered a broken back. Later she moved to Battle Creek, where she joined the Seventh-day Adventist Church. While living there, a young man who sold religious books stayed in her home and often took her for evening carriage rides. His name was Edward Sutherland.

Gotzian not only gave money to Madison, but also to the institutions that today are Portland Adventist Medical Center, Loma Linda University and Paradise Valley Hospital. She eventually moved to Madison, where she was a prominent figure in the school and hospital. She died at the age of 90, with less than $1,000 in her estate. The rest had benefited Adventist healthcare.

Lida Funk Scott also provided much-needed financial assistance. The daughter of Wilfred Funk of the Funk and Wagnall Publishing Company, she once had been a patient at the Battle Creek Sanitarium, and after becoming a Seventh-day Adventist, joined Madison College in 1916. Over the years she donated thousands of dollars to the school and its "rural units." It was she who donated the $30,000 earmarked for Madison to help CME build a hospital in Los Angeles.

One of Madison's purposes was to train students to work in the rural areas where people suffered from poor health, inadequate educational facilities and depleted agricultural land. At one time there were nearly 50 of these "rural units" in Tennessee, Georgia, Mississippi, Alabama, Kentucky and North Carolina.

Madison College and Madison Hospital transferred to denominational ownership in 1963, and the college closed in 1964. The following year the old sanitarium buildings were razed and a replacement facility built. A five-floor patient tower was completed in 1974 and fully staffed by 1981, bringing the hospital's bed capacity to 311. The name was changed to Tennessee Christian Medical Center in 1985.

A 50-bed sister facility known as Highland Hospital—established as Fountain Head Sanitarium in 1929—in nearby Portland became a satellite hospital in 1994. It was renamed Tennessee Christian Medical Center-Portland.

SOURCES

Gish, Ira and Harry Christman, *Madison—God's Beautiful Farm: The E. A. Sutherland Story*, Nampa, Idaho: The Upward Way, 1989.

Hansen, Louis A., *From So Small a Dream*, Nashville, Tennessee: Southern Publishing Association, 1968.

Rittenhouse, Floyd O. Rittenhouse, "E.A. Sutherland, Independent Reformer," *Adventist Heritage*, Winter 1977.

Madison College: School of Divine Origin 1904–1964, Madison College Alumni Association, 1986.

Bryant, Paul A., Komala Dewantara, Eduardo A. Gonzalez, Carol Grannon, Ulrike Hasel, Christina Maria O. Matos, Kenneth E. McHenry, Erling B. Snorrason, Carol Williams; Jerry Moon, instructor, editor, *Edward Alexander Sutherland and Madison College, 1904–1964*, Berrien Springs, Michigan: Andrews University School of Education, 1989.

Chapter 13

Parmele's $9,000 Success Story

Florida Hospital
Established 1908

Escape to Sunshine State

While blizzards blew up North, sanitarium guests spent pleasant winter days in Florida playing croquet, shuffleboard, tennis and golf, watching water birds and alligators in the nearby lake, or relaxing in rocking chairs on the broad porches overlooking Lake Estelle. When winter passed they returned to their northern homes, fleeing the Sunshine State's steamy summers.

Soon after Rufus Wells Parmele moved to Florida in 1907, he began looking for a place to open a health center similar to the other Adventist facilities that now stretched across the United States and overseas. Coming from Nashville, Parmele and his physician wife, Lydia, were well acquainted with the church's early medical work. Before completing her medical training, Lydia had worked as a nurse with her parents in Vicksburg, Mississippi. She was also familiar with Riverside Hospital and the Madison Sanitarium in Tennessee.

The Parmeles found a failed tuberculosis facility that had been developed by a Dr. R.L. Harris at a cost of more than $12,000. Located on 72 acres, the lakeside property included a large frame building, four cottages and a dairy herd. Trees, orange groves, flowering shrubbery and palms enhanced the peaceful setting. Parmele, president of the newly organized Florida Conference of Seventh-day Adventists, offered $9,000 for the property, although the conference had only $4.83 on its books.

When the owner accepted his offer, Parmele turned to local church members to raise the money. They welcomed the opportunity to begin a Battle Creek-style medical work in Central Florida and quickly raised enough money through contributions and stock purchases to avoid incurring debt.

Florida's Turn

"I have no hesitancy in saying that I believe the time has come for Florida to have a sanitarium, so that the light which our sanitariums are established to reflect may shine forth to the people of Florida and to the many health seekers who come from the northern states." —ELLEN WHITE

༜

The 20-bed Florida Sanitarium opened in October 1908, with two physicians, four patients, a nurse and other workers. In time Parmele's $9,000 investment would reap a healthy return for Adventist healthcare, but early growth was hampered by dramatic seasonal fluctuations in population. Florida attracted many wealthy "snowbirds" from the northern states who enjoyed a spa-like winter vacation at the sanitarium, availing themselves of hydrotherapy treatments, massages, healthful diet and recreation. Business was not limited to the resort-type resident, of course. From the beginning, doctors provided acute-care services ranging from surgery to maternity care.

Most organizations experience personnel conflicts of one sort or another, and the young Florida San was no exception. According to author Louis Hansen in *From So Small A Dream*, a serious rift developed between the business manager and medical director around 1929. Among other things, in an effort to avoid malpractice lawsuits, the business manager insisted on being present for all surgeries, which infuriated the physicians. It became virtually impossible to attract new physicians and took several years and personnel changes to remedy the situation.

In the days before air conditioning, summers presented special challenges for the surgical staff. As explained in *Through the Years*, published in 1998 for the hospital's 90th anniversary, "...ceiling and wall-mounted fans provided the only source of cooling.... The surgery rooms were particularly sweltering—the hot surgical lights created immense heat, and the rooms could not be cooled by fans or other devices which might spread dust or particles." Air conditioning was installed in 1958.

Changed Attitude

Martin Andersen didn't think much of the Florida Sanitarium and Hospital in the early 1950s. As editor, and later owner and publisher, of the "Orlando Sentinel," *he refused to print anything about the hospital in the newspaper.*

Homer Grove, public relations director at the time, arranged for Andersen to receive free physical therapy treatments. He accepted the

invitation, and in time came to appreciate the hospital staff. After a while he began bringing them copies of the newspaper, and also gave orchids to new mothers. And, yes, he told Grove he would print whatever he brought to the newspaper. This went on for more than 10 years. Andersen even arranged to build a house on the hospital property so he could live there in his final years.

Over time he and his wife, Gracia, donated millions of dollars to the hospital, and a number of facilities are named in their honor, including a garden and orchid room, the Martin Andersen wing at Florida Hospital Orlando and the Martin Andersen Cancer Center at Florida Hospital Altamonte.

With the 1960s came an important period in the history of Central Florida—and consequently for Adventist healthcare. These were boom years for tourism and business, and under Don Welch's administration from 1961 to 1973, the hospital made its final transition from a sanitarium to a modern acute-care hospital.

One of his first hurdles was a medical staff that had little interest in growing, in either quality or quantity. As a result, the 34-year-old administrator took some tough stands to upgrade the staff and attract additional board-certified physicians.

Welch believed that Adventist healthcare had the opportunity to improve its mission of quality care and service in Central Florida. It could become a leader—or risk being left behind while other hospitals marched in step with the rapidly growing community. Big changes were occurring in the healthcare industry and the timing was right for Florida Hospital.

During the Welch years the hospital grew from 160 to 474 patient beds, and initiated such services and programs as the region's first intensive-care unit, a cardiac-care unit, cardiac catheterization and open-heart surgery, the nation's first orthopedic "clean air surgery," a family practice residency program and an organ transplant program. Welch also bought a large pasture north of Orlando, and in 1973 opened a 104-bed satellite facility called Florida Hospital Altamonte. Today it is a 278-bed hospital.

A System Begins

From time to time, Florida Hospital received requests to open hospitals in other communities or to manage existing hospitals. But there was no organizational mechanism for such arrangements. Seeing what was happening throughout the healthcare industry, Welch and other Adventist leaders recognized that the church's many small stand-alone hospitals must be part of larger systems that could provide strong management expertise, centralization of certain services and the benefits of economies of scale. With this in mind, Welch left Florida Hospital in 1973 to devote his attention to pioneering the organization that is today's Adventist Health System.

Bob Scott followed Welch as president of Florida Hospital, and it continued to flourish. Some of the advances made between 1973 and 1979 include a 48-bed pediatric unit, 40-bed heart unit and 65-bed orthopedic unit at the Orlando campus, and a 7-bed coronary-care unit at Altamonte. Also during this time the 50-bed hospital in Apopka, a town north of Orlando, became the second Florida Hospital satellite.

Mardian Blair came from Portland Adventist Hospital and the Northwest Medical Foundation in Oregon to serve as Florida Hospital president from 1979 to 1984. Among other projects, he oversaw the development of the Florida Heart Institute, the opening of a level II neonatal unit, an 80-bed expansion of the Altamonte satellite, and a $120 million construction project that included a medical office building, freestanding psychiatric center, and a patient tower that increased the Orlando facility's capacity to 849 beds.

Big Plans

The GC and Union treasurers had their annual meeting in Orlando just as plans for this expansion were being finalized. Mardian Blair invited us to come to the hospital one evening for a presentation. We were impressed with the plans but very nervous about the $120 million price tag. It proved to be the right thing to do at that time. —WILLIAM MURRILL, RETIRED UNDERTREASURER, GENERAL CONFERENCE OF SEVENTH-DAY ADVENTISTS

In 1984 Welch was appointed president of what turned out to be a short-lived national Adventist health system. Blair was named president of what was then called Adventist Health System/Sunbelt, consisting of the Adventist hospitals in the church's Southern and Southwestern unions. Tom Werner took over the helm of Florida Hospital, and led the organization through 16 years of tremendous growth in services, patient capacity, acquisitions and community relationships.

Some of the projects completed during the Werner years include a center for women's medicine, Martin Andersen Cancer Pavilion at Altamonte, Florida Hospital College of Health Sciences, the Walt Disney Memorial Cancer Institute, a state-of-the-art surgical wing, the opening of Celebration Health—a healthy community model and showcase for medical skills, equipment, technology and education—in the planned community of Celebration, and the opening of RDV Sportsplex, a joint venture between the hospital and the parent corporation of the Orlando Magic basketball team.

Large Adventist hospitals have helped small ones ever since the days of the Battle Creek Sanitarium in the 1800s. This is certainly true of Florida Hospital. In the early years of Adventist Health System, Florida Hospital supported virtually all of the church's hospitals in the southern and southwestern United States until they either became financially viable or were divested. Without Florida Hospital's support, some of today's strong Adventist hospitals would not have had a chance to grow and thrive.

Meanwhile, Florida Hospital continued to enlarge its service area. The satellite concept begun during the Welch years laid the foundation for the Orlando-based hospital to expand to multiple campuses. In 1990 the stand-alone Orlando General Hospital in East Orlando needed a strong parent organization in order to secure managed care contracts. A merger with Florida Hospital made that possible. In 1992 Waterman Memorial Hospital in Lake County recognized its future depended on becoming part of a large organization, and chose to unite with Florida Hospital. Both Orlando General and Waterman were gifts to Florida Hospital.

In 1993 the acquisition of a small hospital in Kissimmee expanded Florida Hospital's market to Osceola County. Working with the planned community of Celebration, in 1997 Florida Hospital opened a second hospital in Osceola County, the innovative Celebration Health. With the purchase of the 334-bed Winter Park Memorial Hospital in 2000, Florida Hospital now has a total of seven campuses, making it the largest private, not-for-profit hospital and second largest hospital overall in the state. It is a recognized leader in cardiology, cancer treatment, psychiatry, women's medicine, obstetrics and pediatrics, neuroscience, orthopedics, organ transplantation, limb replantation and sports medicine.

Today all Adventist Health System hospitals in Florida are under the umbrella of the Florida Division, and several bear the Florida Hospital name while remaining separate legal entities. Altogether there are 17 Adventist hospital campuses in nine counties: Orange, Seminole, Osceola, Lake, Volusia, Flagler, Highlands, Hardee and Pasco. When current expansion and replacement projects are completed, the Florida Division will represent approximately 3,000 patient beds.

Health System of Choice

Five Florida hospitals became part of the Adventist Health System family in 2000. Among these were the three hospitals of Memorial Health

Systems, a community-owned not-for-profit organization based in Ormond Beach.

Over the years leaders from Memorial Health Systems and Adventist Health System had developed a high regard for their respective emphases on quality. When it became evident that its future depended on a close relationship with a large successful organization, Memorial chose Adventist Health System, in part for its spiritual mission.

Although Memorial was not a church-affiliated organization, the owners believed the Christian mission closely matched their values and goals. Trusting the Adventists to continue what the community had begun with these hospitals, the owners transferred ownership of Memorial Health Systems to Adventist Health System. The merger of these facilities, valued at $175 million less liabilities, is the largest single gift to any organization of the Seventh-day Adventist Church.

These are the Florida Division facilities as of December 2000, with the present number of patient beds: Florida Hospital (Orlando campus) (902 beds); FH Heartland Medical Center (101 beds); FH Altamonte (278 beds); FH Apopka (50 beds); East Pasco Medical Center (139 beds); FH Lake Placid (50 beds); FH East Orlando (123 beds); FH Waterman (182 beds); FH Kissimmee (40 beds); FH Wauchula (50 beds); FH Fish Memorial (97 beds); FH Celebration Health (60 beds); Memorial Hospital-Flagler (81 beds); Memorial Hospital-Ormond Beach (205 beds); Memorial Hospital-Peninsula (119-beds); Florida Hospital DeLand (156 beds); Winter Park Memorial Hospital (334 beds)

SOURCES

"Florida Hospital: 75 Years of Care. 75 Years of Caring," 1983.

Hansen, Louis A., *From So Small a Dream*, Nashville, Tennessee: Southern Publishing Association, 1968.

Norman, R. Steven III, "Edson White's Southern Work Remembered," *Southern Tidings*, February 2001.

Howes, Melinda, *Florida Hospital: Through the Years*, Orlando, Florida: Florida Hospital, 1998.

Interviews and Notes: Rich Rainer and William Murrill.

Chapter 14

The Lord Would Be Pleased

Park Ridge Hospital
Established 1910

Blue Ridge Mountain Retreat

In the early days patients came by horse and buggy or wagon, and later by train. They stayed in individual cottages where meals and medications were delivered to them. Sometime in 1927 a larger building was completed with a long porch where patients could enjoy the peaceful views and surroundings of the Blue Ridge Mountains.

Adventist healthcare in North Carolina began with a conversation between two women near Asheville one evening in 1909. Ellen White had stopped in Asheville while traveling by train from Tennessee, to a meeting of church leaders in Washington, D.C. Ever since the end of the Civil War, she had urged farmers, builders, teachers and missionaries to move to the South, but few had responded.

After speaking to a group of church members in Asheville, Mrs. White stayed in the home of Martha Rumbough. The wife of an inventor and daughter of a manufacturer, Rumbough had generously shared her wealth to establish churches in the region. On that evening in 1909 she mentioned that she would like to give additional help. Mrs. White was ready for her offer.

"The Lord would be pleased if you would start a medical and educational work in the vicinity of Asheville," she said.

Two men played an important part in establishing a school and medical work in this area. One was Arthur Whitefield Spalding, author and teacher formerly from Emmanuel Missionary College in Michigan. He was selling and writing books and trying to recruit others to western North Carolina. The second man was Professor Sidney Brownsberger, teacher, administrator and minister. He had purchased a small farm where he and his wife lived with their three children.

Spalding accepted responsibility for finding a location for the proposed work in the Asheville area. Mrs. White had specified that it must be a country setting with a good supply of water and timber, available soil and access to roads and railways. There should also be some buildings on the property. While selling books one day, he learned of a rundown place known as Byers' Plantation, and he set out to find it.

It Had Potential

"The road was winding, and dusty and long until he topped a hill. He stood where the road crossed the old Indian trading path known as the Howard Gap Road, and looked down into a valley.... [The old plantation] had been worked since 1798. The topsoil had eroded, and deep red gullies ribboned the area near the dilapidated old barn. The two-story farmhouse dated from 1885 and was in great need of repairs. Weeds and brush were everywhere. But into Spalding's poetic mind came recollections of the words, 'As the mountains are round about Jerusalem' (Psalm 125:2, KJV), and he knew this was the place he was searching for." —MOUNTAIN MEMORIES

According to the deed dated March 11, 1910, the Adventists purchased 416 acres for $5,750. The trustees named in the deed were Martha E. Rumbough, Edward A. Sutherland, R.L. Williams, Percy T. Magan and Sidney Brownsberger.

This was the beginning of today's Fletcher Academy and Park Ridge Hospital. With the construction of a cottage with two treatment rooms in 1916, Adventists built the first healthcare facility for the mountain people of western North Carolina, for many years known as the Mountain Sanitarium.

Brownsberger's son and daughter, John and Ethel Brownsberger, both Madison College graduates, were the first nurses at the Mountain San and the first registered nurses in North Carolina. In 1920 John married Elsie Peterson, a young woman he had proposed to at Madison College in 1914. Amazingly, they had seen each other only twice during the six years that lapsed between the proposal and the wedding. John and another nurse, Forrest Bliss, studied medicine at the College of Medical Evangelists in California, and returned to work at the Mountain San.

The authors of *Mountain Memories* record the following account of the Brownsberger's dedicated service.

Devoted Couple Serve Fletcher

After the untimely death of two daughters in 1929, John and Elsie "buried themselves in the work of developing the Hospital and School of Nursing at Fletcher. John worked untiringly during the depression years, many times getting paid in farm produce or labor, as money was scarce. He often would be called out at night to travel over muddy mountain roads to see patients. He never complained except once when he arrived at a remote farmhouse at 2 a.m. to discover that his patient was a sick cow! He did all types of surgery during those years, and obstetrics—many times giving the anesthetic as well. It was during this time that he helped to establish the Blue Shield Insurance Plan for North Carolina...."

Another name closely linked to the history of the Mountain San is Lelia Patterson, who devoted her life to the health needs of the mountain people. A registered nurse from the Hinsdale Sanitarium near Chicago, she moved to Asheville in 1919 to help start a vegetarian cafeteria and treatment room. That facility, called Good Health Place, merged with the Mountain San in 1920 and Patterson began a 43-year affiliation with the hospital.

True Mountain Missionary

When she died in 1975, Leila Patterson left a legacy of compassionate care and a pioneer spirit that was the hallmark of many early Adventist healthcare workers. In the early days she traveled by Model-T Ford over unpaved mountain roads around Asheville to treat the sick and deliver babies. Her services were available to all regardless of color, creed or ability to pay. She took food and clothing to those in need and used her own money to help pay their hospital bills. Through her Good Neighbor Clubs, she taught people how to grow their own food, prepare nutritious meals and improve family health.

The sanitarium operated a school of nursing for 56 years. Its graduates were highly sought by hospitals all over the country, as well as for overseas service.

The name of the Mountain San was changed to Fletcher Hospital around 1973. It became part of Adventist Health System/Sunbelt Health Care Corporation in 1984. The name was changed to Park Ridge Hospital in 1985, and the present facility opened in 1986. The former hospital plant now houses a long-term-care facility operated by Adventist Care Centers, a division of Adventist Health System.

SOURCES

Mountain Memories: The Story of Mountain Sanitarium and Hospital School of Nursing, Collegedale, Tennessee: The College Press, undated.

"Lelia Patterson Center: Doorway to Lifestyle Enhancement," (fund-raising publication), Fletcher, North Carolina: Fletcher Academy, undated.

Chapter 15

Training Center in the City

White Memorial Medical Center
Established 1913

Turning Point

A gentle knock interrupted a crucial meeting of church officials and leaders of the College of Medical Evangelists at Loma Linda, California, in 1915. Despite all the hard work of school leaders, the school had received only a C rating—the lowest granted by the American Medical Association's accrediting agency. The men gathered that day were deciding the future of the young school. Who would dare interrupt such an important meeting?

Someone opened the door to find four women requesting admittance. Josephine Gotzian was a woman of means who had contributed generously to the Madison Sanitarium and Hospital, Paradise Valley Sanitarium, Portland Sanitarium and Hospital and other places. Hetty Haskell was a teacher and wife of the popular evangelist Stephen Haskell—a woman known for her faith and belief in the power of the Word of God. Her widowed sister, Emma Gray, was a person with more faith than money, but had a history of overcoming great obstacles in her lifetime. Dr. Florence Keller of the Glendale Sanitarium had been a physician with her husband in New Zealand.

These women—sent by Dr. Percy Magan's friend, Dr. Edward Sutherland, in Tennessee—had something to say. (See Chapter 12 on Tennessee Christian Medical Center.) *They asked that the school be allowed to continue, with a teaching hospital built in Los Angeles to house the clinical division. Further, the hospital should be dedicated to the memory of Ellen White, who had recently died. The men were not to worry about the money for the hospital. They should leave that in the hands of the women of the church. Needless to say, the men were speechless. Magan later said a "sacred hush pervaded the room" as the women thanked the men for their courtesy and left.*

&

74

The White Memorial Medical Center actually began as an outpatient clinic in 1913 to provide part of the clinical experience needed by students at the College of Medical Evangelists (CME). (See Chapter 9 on Loma Linda University Medical Center.) In 1915 the school had a choice of either expanding its clinical program or closing.

While some thought the time had come to close the school, others believed Adventists had a medical mission that required fully qualified physicians. The vote was taken to continue the four-year program and build a teaching facility in Los Angeles.

The school bought a block of property in the Boyle Heights area near the Los Angeles County Hospital, where CME students were already receiving some of their clinical training. The first cottages comprising White Memorial Hospital opened in January 1918, with additional bungalows built as money became available. Eventually "The White," as it became known, consisted of nine buildings filling the entire block.

Hectic workdays in Los Angeles were a sharp contrast to the tranquil sanitarium life in rural Loma Linda. In the first 10 years of operation the clinic averaged 71,000 patients per year, more than any other outpatient facility in the city. Contracts with a railroad company, the Los Angeles police and fire departments and the Ascot Speedway helped fund the large amount of charity care The White provided.

In addition to working in the clinic, student nurses and medical students also made "home deliveries" throughout East Los Angeles. This was called "Outside OB," which often required middle-of-the-night trips by streetcar to assist women delivering their babies at home. These experiences produced many interesting stories, some of which may have strayed slightly from the truth in the retelling over the years. Maxine Atteberry related the following in her history of the Loma Linda University School of Nursing:

Slippery Situation

"An inept medical student had delivered his first baby. When he tried to lift the infant by the feet as he had seen done, it slipped through his fingers and fell to the floor. He picked it up, fortunately unhurt and squalling lustily. When he looked up he was facing the disapproving eyes of the baby's grandmother. Having a presence of mind which far exceeded his manual dexterity he quickly said, 'He's a fine baby, Ma'am. We sometimes have to drop 'em two or three times to make 'em cry.'"

Erwin Remboldt, first president of Adventist Health Services (Adventist Health), was The White's administrator/president for a total of

10 years. He arrived in 1950 fresh from Union College in Lincoln, Nebraska. With a new business degree, he says he expected to get "a fairly reasonable job." Instead, he had to get up at 5 a.m. to post the patient ledger.

"I didn't even know how to run an adding machine," he says.

After a few months he was appointed assistant accountant, and later personnel director. Then one day the dean at Loma Linda offered to send him to school for an advanced degree in hospital administration.

"It was an opportunity I couldn't refuse," says Remboldt. "I thought an angel had just dropped from heaven."

After completing his degree at the University of Chicago, he returned to The White for an internship in 1955.

"They gave me a little office, but I really didn't have an awful lot to do," he recalls.

That situation changed within a few months when the board elected him administrator, a position he held until 1960 when he went to Glendale. Within four years he would be administrator of both facilities.

Quick Work

Ray Pelton arrived at The White as administrator in 1960, only three months before a review by the Joint Commission on Accreditation of Healthcare Organizations. Discovering 3,000 incomplete patient charts, he began pressuring the staff to update them. While all were not finished before the inspection, the accreditation was renewed based on the amount of work accomplished in three months' time. When Pelton moved to the New England Sanitarium and Hospital in 1963, discussions of consolidating The White and Loma Linda campuses had already begun.

The two-campus medical school had never been ideal. In 1951 the Council on Medical Education had strongly recommended that the school consolidate campuses. It took the board of trustees nearly two years to agree, and several more years passed before the consolidation actually happened.

In question was whether the school should be in Los Angeles or Loma Linda. Studies were commissioned and arguments went on for about nine years before a decision was made in 1962. Shortly after Dr. David Hinshaw became dean, the matter went to the church's Annual Council in Washington, D.C., which voted for Loma Linda.

Many who thought the school should move to Loma Linda also thought the Los Angeles facility should be sold. They didn't believe it could survive without the medical school. However, The White had been part of the Los Angeles community for more than 50 years, and more was at stake than loss of a hospital. The local Adventist community was one of the largest, most prosperous and influential in Southern California.

Cree Sandefur, president of the church's Southern California Conference, called Remboldt at nearby Glendale Sanitarium and Hospital, and they agreed to ask the Loma Linda board not to sell The White. The board agreed, and on January 1, 1964, the hospital was renamed White Memorial Medical Center. Sandefur asked Remboldt to be administrator.

"But I'm administrator at Glendale," he protested.

Sandefur persuaded him to take both hospitals and divide his time between them.

Uncertain Future

"We had no money at The White," Remboldt recalls. "We figured we needed about $4 million for operating capital."

Remboldt and Sandefur went to the Security Pacific Bank in Glendale, which handled accounts for the Glendale Sanitarium, the Southern California Conference of Seventh-day Adventists and the church's Pacific Union Conference. They met with a Mr. Dewer, who listened politely and asked several questions about the hospital's financial situation.

The two men had to admit they didn't know whether the hospital would make it financially, and probably were not too surprised when Dewer said he could not loan them $4 million. However, Sandefur was prepared with a response.

"If this bank cannot loan us the money, we will have to pull the accounts of the Glendale San, the Southern California Conference and the Pacific Union Conference, too," he said.

Dewer excused himself and returned shortly with the loan approved.

When Remboldt went to The White in 1964, it was losing about half a million dollars a year. It was in a low-income part of Los Angeles, the medical staff needed reorganization, and two floors had been closed due of a lack of nurses. At that time the hospital paid nurses about $150 below the average community rate, and Remboldt knew he had to increase their salaries. However, in those days wages for all Adventist hospital employees were based on a ministerial salary. Remboldt spent two days at church headquarters in Washington, D.C., persuading officials to allow him to raise his nurses' salaries. They finally agreed to an additional $10 a month.

However, it took more than a $10 raise to recruit the nurses for The White. Remboldt and his administrative team spent a lot of time on their knees, praying that the Lord would help them find personnel. After about four months he had enough nurses to staff the vacant floors.

Every week it seemed that a physician or key employee moved to Loma Linda. Fortunately, the remaining medical staff rallied to support the needs of the local community and turn the place around. Among other things, this meant eliminating the part-pay operation of the clinic. The White also received Hill-Burton funding to replace the old clinic and add a medical office building. Slowly the hospital began to breathe on its own, and within a year it was breaking even financially. Remboldt remained president of The White and Glendale until 1968, at which time he went back to Glendale full time. He returned to The White for a short time in 1983.

White Memorial continued to grow. However, 1987 brought a financial crisis that threatened to end its long history. A turnaround finally occurred when the state began providing money to hospitals with a high number of Medi-Cal and indigent patients.

Modern-day Miracles

A consultant I had known when he headed Medi-Cal called to tell me Senate Bill 855 was within days of coming up for a vote. It meant millions of state and federal dollars would go to government teaching hospitals and children's hospitals that care for a high number of Medi-Cal and indigent patients. With only some minor modifications, it could include some other hospitals that met certain qualifications for these "disproportionate share funds." My friend estimated it could mean $10 million to $12 million a year for White Memorial.

I immediately called Harvey Rudisaile, then president of The White, and told him to see our good friends at the Los Angeles County Hospital who were spearheading the bill. He went over there, got to the right people right away, and in no time enlisted their support for changing the bill.

Meanwhile, I telephoned a very prominent attorney in Los Angeles—the main legal counsel for some of the large for-profit hospitals. Miraculously, I reached him on the first call, and he agreed to work with us. Then I called all my friends at the Catholic and Lutheran hospitals in Los Angeles. Again, I got all of them on the first call. I called the California Healthcare Association, and reached the president on the first call.

Adrian Zytkoskee in the corporate office also made some important calls. It was a mammoth undertaking in a very short period of time.

Within a couple of days, we sat down with the consultant and attorney to make the changes that would widen the net of hospitals eligible for these funds. The bill passed with our changes. To this day, I have a copy of the first million-dollar check to White Memorial Medical Center. (Loma Linda University Medical Center and Paradise Valley Hospital also have benefited from SB 855.)

In addition to these funds, White Memorial Medical Center has qualified for nearly $100 million to rebuild as a result of a FEMA earthquake preparedness program following the Northridge earthquake of 1994. —FRANK DUPPER, RETIRED PRESIDENT AND CEO, ADVENTIST HEALTH

Today the 350-bed White Memorial Medical Center is a successful full-service hospital providing quality and comprehensive inpatient and outpatient services in the tradition of health, healing and Christian compassion.

SOURCES

Atteberry, Maxine, *From Pinafores to Pantsuits*: *The Story of Loma Linda University School of Nursing*, Loma Linda, California, 1975.

Herber, Raymond, editor, *The Department of Medicine from 1909 to 2000*, Loma Linda, California: Department of Medicine, School of Medicine of Loma Linda University, 1999.

Johns, Warren L., and Richard H. Utt, editors, *The Vision Bold*, Washington, D.C.: Review and Herald Publishing Association, 1977.

Judd, Wayne, tape recorded interviews with Don Ammon, Frank Dupper and Erwin Remboldt, 1998.

Interviews: Frank Dupper, Ray Pelton and Erwin Remboldt.

Chapter 16

Mother D's Promise

Riverside Sanitarium and Hospital
1927–1983

One Woman's Commitment

When word spread around Nashville's white community that Nellie Druillard was organizing some kind of colony for black folks, they complained about her project for the "Nigras," but she could not be swayed. She bought the property, contributed the money to build Riverside Sanitarium, paid the bills when patient census was low and single-handedly managed the infant institution.

The roots of Riverside Hospital trace back to the late 1800s when Edson White sailed the Mississippi River with a band of volunteers on a steamer called *Morning Star.* Stopping wherever they could find an audience to listen to their Bible studies and health lectures, they laid the groundwork for Adventist healthcare in the South.

Ellen White published several appeals in the church paper, *Review and Herald,* to help the emancipated African-Americans in the South. Both whites and blacks responded, some at the urging of their teacher Dr. John Harvey Kellogg at Battle Creek. One of these was Dr. Lottie C. Isbell.

Any work for the African-Americans in the South at this time was difficult, and anyone coming from the North was regarded with skepticism, if not disdain. This was certainly true for Isbell, the first black Seventh-day Adventist physician. She went to Nashville in 1902 to work with Fred and Fannie Young, who had been there about a year. Isbell was not prepared for the competition she found among medical facilities in Nashville. As Louis Reynolds records in *We Have Tomorrow*, the city already had four medical schools offering free services, a large free city hospital and around 60 African-American doctors. This community had no use for a fledgling operation promoting the "rag treatments" of hydrotherapy.

As a result, Isbell left Nashville and moved to Huntsville, Alabama, in 1905 to be resident physician at Oakwood, an Adventist school established for African-Americans in 1896. She also worked with J. Jim Pearson, another Battle Creek graduate, who operated a small sanitarium in Birmingham.

Segregated Clientele

Pearson's treatment facility for white clientele was immediately successful, attracting senators and representatives, lawyers and judges. Non-white clientele had to be served at night, because Birmingham's segregation laws would not permit him to serve blacks "except at night with the shades tightly drawn."

During this time Isbell married David Blake, a Jamaican minister, who returned with her to Tennessee in 1908 to set up treatment rooms again. The following year they established the Rock City Sanitarium. Blake was a pastor and also had completed the medical course at Meharry Medical School. The couple struggled in vain to make the sanitarium venture succeed, but in 1912 they finally went to Panama as missionaries.

It would take someone with money to support a medical work for Nashville's African-American population. Nellie Druillard was a woman of means with a keen business head. She had served as treasurer and/or auditor in church organizations in the United States and in South Africa, where she and her husband worked for six years. Affectionately known as "Mother D," she helped several Adventist organizations, including Emmanuel Missionary College (now Andrews University), Madison College, Madison Sanitarium (now Tennessee Christian Medical Center) and several self-supporting ventures such as Pearson's.

Promise Remembered

Druillard once promised Mrs. White that she would build a sanitarium for the African-Americans of the South. As she became involved in Emmanuel Missionary College and the Madison organizations, that promise was laid aside. Unfortunately, she was injured when a car struck her in San Francisco. But, while recovering from her injuries, she pledged to keep her promise for the African-Americans.

From her personal funds Druillard spent approximately $250,000 to build cottages, equip the hospital, and operate the sanitarium and nursing program. She also trained about 80 practical nurses. When she could no longer manage the hospital herself, in 1935 she gave Riverside Sanitarium to the General Conference of Seventh-day Adventists.

Many others played important roles in Riverside's history, but as with any institution, a few stand above the rest.

Chaney Johnson

After hearing of Druillard's experience, Chaney Johnson quit her $150-a-month position with a physician, and joined the Riverside Sanitarium for $20 a month. Sometimes she didn't receive even that much. In fact, for two and a half years she accepted no salary. Whenever she needed a dress, shoes, toothpaste or other necessities, someone seemed to provide exactly what she needed at just the right time. In later years she said those were the happiest days of her life.

Johnson was well known by some of the hospital's wealthy and influential clientele, who raved about her meatless recipes traditionally prepared with pork. One professor mentioned this during a speaking engagement at which she was present.

"If anybody had told me you could prepare beans without meat, I'd never have believed them," he said. "You know, Seventh-day Adventists are clever people. They can make the best soybean pork chops you've ever eaten."

Riverside's first two business managers were Harry and Louis Ford, who came from Hinsdale Sanitarium near Chicago. After Druillard gave Riverside to the church, Harry Ford was asked to manage it. This he did only until 1938, when cancer cut short his life of service.

Louis Ford followed his brother as manager for the next six years, working with a meager budget and staff. His wife and father also worked at the hospital, usually without pay. Ford did anything that needed to be done. He bought groceries, transported patients, cared for the garden, helped in physiotherapy and even repaired tractors.

Dr. Carl Dent

For more than 25 years the name Dr. Carl Dent was synonymous with Riverside. A 1939 graduate of the College of Medical Evangelists (Loma Linda University), he was the first black intern at the Los Angeles County Hospital. In Nashville, he set up a small clinic across the street from Riverside Hospital where people lined up to see him every day. It didn't matter that he had few helpers or lacked the latest in technology. Patients loved Dent. In fact, one woman who became ill while traveling in

Europe returned all the way back to Nashville to make sure Dr. Dent took care of her.

Except for about six years, the doctor served at Riverside his whole career. Loyal to the church and its medical mission, he helped recruit 66 doctors to the South.

❧

Despite valiant efforts by these pioneers and many other people who worked hard to keep Riverside viable, the hospital ultimately failed to produce sufficient funds to continue its mission. It closed in 1983.

SOURCES

Dent, Carl A., M.D., "I Expect a Miracle," *The North American Regional Voice*, 1983.

Justiss, Jacob, *Angels in Ebony*, Toledo, Ohio: Jet Printing Services, 1975.

Reynolds, Louis B., "Riverside: A Medical Ministry Begun in Nashville," *The North American Regional Voice,* 1983.

Reynolds, Louis B., *We Have Tomorrow*, Washington, D.C.: Review and Herald Publishing Association, 1984.

Rucker, Womack H., Jr., "The Crisis, The Solution," *The North American Regional Voice,* 1983.

Chapter 17

Influence of a Surgeon's Prayer

Takoma Adventist Hospital
Established 1928

Unexpected Invitation

After finishing an internship at White Memorial Hospital in Los Angeles in 1960, Dr. James Ray McKinney went home to Morristown, Tennessee, for a little vacation before returning for a surgery residency. One day while he was home, R.E. Crawford from the Georgia-Cumberland Conference of Seventh-day Adventists came to see him.

"Dr. Coolidge is 71 years old, and he's sitting up there in Greeneville with no help. That's why I've come to see you—to ask you to go up there and work with him at Takoma Hospital," Crawford said.

"I can't do that," McKinney replied. "I'm going back to California."

Crawford pleaded for the young man to drive 30 miles to Greeneville and just talk with Coolidge, which McKinney finally agreed to do. He knew Coolidge was a good surgeon—a Fellow in the American College of Surgeons and the International College of Surgeons. When he was a boy, McKinney's mother had taken him to Coolidge.

The older doctor had started the hospital in the 1920s, and in 1960 he was still captain of the ship. However, the time had come to turn it over to a younger person. He asked McKinney to do it for one year—which turned into more than 41 years.

After working six years in a Pennsylvania mining community, Dr. LeRoy Coolidge recognized this was not what he wanted in life. He moved to Washington, D.C., where he had gone to medical school, and joined the staff of the Washington Sanitarium in Takoma Park, Maryland. There he worked with Dr. Harry Miller, who had a profound influence on him. (See Chapter 24 on China.)

Takoma Park Connection

In the early 1920s some affluent patients from Greene County, Tennessee, were traveling to the Washington San for healthcare services. They had learned about the facility through one of Miller's patients. The man had been extremely depressed and was considering suicide when Miller told him he needed a portion of his colon removed. Figuring he would never live through surgery, he agreed to the operation.

Miller offered his usual prayer before surgery, unaware that the patient expected to die. As it turned out, the man not only recovered, but his whole outlook on life changed—largely the result of hearing the physician's prayer. Feeling better than ever, the man told his family and friends in Tennessee about his experience. Soon they were also going to the Washington San. Eventually someone talked with Miller and his colleague, Dr. Daniel Kress, about opening a sanitarium in Greeneville.

Miller and Kress each had been pioneer missionaries—Miller in China, and Kress with his physician wife, Lauretta, in England, Australia and New Zealand. The two men traveled to Tennessee where they were duly impressed with the quiet community in Greene County. But the people here would have to wait for a sanitarium.

Meanwhile, in 1923 Roy Bowen and his wife, both graduate nurses, set up hydrotherapy rooms and a vegetarian cafeteria in a large house on Main Street. Miller and Coolidge went there three times in 1925 to do surgeries. Coolidge then moved to Greeneville, and in 1926 bought the facility, which was called Branch Takoma Park Sanitarium. Two registered nurses from the Washington San came to help him.

Another nurse, Virgil Robert Bottomley, also from the Washington San, was Coolidge's right-hand man from 1926 to 1941, doing just about anything that needed to be done, from bookkeeping to X-rays. At age 41 he enrolled in medical school at the University of Tennessee at Memphis, and returning to Greeneville, admitted patients to Takoma Hospital for many years.

A school of nursing was started in 1926. Interestingly, the student uniforms were modeled after those used at Walter Reed Army Hospital where Coolidge's sisters studied in Washington, D.C. The Takoma school trained registered nurses for 20 years. It changed to a practical nursing program in 1946, and at one time offered a "missionary nurse" course. Coolidge considered nursing to be "a profession based on sacrifice and service," and was pleased that many Takoma graduates became overseas missionaries.

When the Main Street facility became inadequate, 24 community leaders organized a corporation and each invested at least $1,000. One donated land to build a three-story 40-bed hospital, which opened January 1, 1928. Coolidge gradually bought out the stockholders, and in 1954 deeded the hospital to the Southern Union Conference of Seventh-day Adventists.

As founder, owner and medical director, Coolidge had the first and last word regarding the hospital as long as he was associated with it. Twenty-six-year-old McKinney joined him in 1960.

"He kind of adopted me as his son," says McKinney. "For 10 years I stood under him and he taught me surgery."

The younger doctor knew if the hospital was to be successful some changes must be made. The physical plant was outdated, and nothing was being done diagnostically in X-ray or lab.

"I called Don Rees, president of the Southern Union, and told him, 'You've got to send me some help if I'm going to make this place survive,'" McKinney recalls.

Rees asked Don Welch, the new administrator at the Florida Sanitarium and Hospital in Orlando, to go to Greeneville and see what he could do. Although Welch and McKinney were both from Tennessee, they had never met.

Spruced-up Hospital

"Don came up here and we formed a finance committee, and we started spending money. We upgraded the plant. We put in new lighting. We put in a new entrance. We put in new carpet. We bought new laboratory equipment and hired new staff. Don came up here every three months for about five years. He had grown up at Madison, which was based on the idea of a large hospital helping all these little hospitals. So, at the same time he was building up Florida Hospital, he started helping in other places, and he began to see that a health system would benefit the church's hospitals." —DR. JAMES RAY MCKINNEY

After seven years at Takoma, McKinney finally saw the medical staff grow by two more CME graduates. Dr. John Shaw had moved to Greeneville when he was a teen. After completing medical school and a stint with the United States Navy, he returned to Takoma—along with his friend Dr. Michael Odell. They have been on the medical staff since 1968. At age 80 Coolidge stopped practicing medicine and moved from Greeneville, leaving the hospital in the hands of a capable young staff.

Charter Board Member

While attending an Annual Council of Adventist church leaders in the early 1970s, McKinney watched Welch writing names on the back of an envelope.

"I'm forming a new board, and I think you could help," Welch said.

"Well, Don, if you think I could help, I'd be happy to do it," McKinney said.

The list on the envelope was the beginning of the first board of directors for Adventist Health System/Sunbelt Healthcare Corporation, formed in 1973. Takoma Adventist Hospital was among the church-operated facilities to became part of that organization. McKinney served on the board until April 2001. He was also on the board of Adventist Health System/US during the four years it existed, 1985–1989.

When Takoma Adventist Hospital needed a new president in late 1992, McKinney was surprised to receive a phone call from his friend Welch, then president of Huguley Memorial Medical Center in Texas.

"I hear you don't have a president at Takoma," Welch said.

"That's right," McKinney said.

Welch said he'd like the position.

"Don, would you come?" McKinney was ecstatic.

Welch planned to work two more years before retiring and wanted to spend them at Takoma. He and his wife, Jean, owned a home in Greeneville. It was several miles from town and they had to drive through a cemetery and across a brook to reach it. They moved to Greeneville in December 1992, planning to live there for many years.

A Pioneer Dies

One day Welch approached his physician friend. "J. R., I've got a terrible pain in my abdomen that's been bothering me for about a week," he said.

The doctor ordered a CAT scan, which revealed a large retroperitoneal mass.

"Everybody knew the moment they saw it that it was a lymphoma," said McKinney.

After 22 months of treatment at Florida Hospital and Duke University Medical Center in North Carolina, he died on October 7, 1997. Sometime before his death, Welch had told his wife he wanted McKinney to have the sermon and eulogy at his funeral. His other request was to be buried in the cemetery near their country home.

For 75 years, an Adventist hospital and a team of dedicated physicians, nurses and other staff have served the residents of Greene County, Tennessee. It is likely that none of this would have happened had it not been for a surgeon's prayer many years ago and many miles away, in a place called Takoma Park.

SOURCES

Coolidge, L.E., "Founder Relates History of Takoma Hospital and Sanitarium," *The Greeneville Sun*, May 11, 1948, reprinted in Takoma Adventist Hospital's 60 anniversary brochure, 1988.

Moore, Raymond S., *China Doctor*, Mt. View, California: Pacific Press Publishing Association, *1969*.

Interview: Dr. James Ray McKinney.

Chapter 18

Forty-five Cent Refund

Porter Adventist Hospital
Established 1930

Overpayment Returned

"Dear Sir: Your letter of 10th with [a] check for 45 cents received, and I thank you for it and return it to you for credit [to] your general fund. I feel I have underpaid you all for your kind and careful treatment and attention, and I owe you all a debt of gratitude for the kind consideration while with you. Mrs. Porter and I are well, and I am gaining strength daily. With our regards and best wishes to you all." —HENRY M. PORTER

Denver businessman Henry Porter sometimes spent winters with his daughter in Southern California. On one of these visits in 1903, he came down with a cold, and she suggested that he go to Glendale Sanitarium for a hydrotherapy treatment. He found it so relaxing that he fell asleep on the treatment table. When he tried to give his therapist a one-dollar tip, the young man said the sanitarium paid him and it wouldn't be right to accept a tip, too. Porter would not forget that young employee's integrity.

About 25 years later, while staying near San Diego, Porter again came down with a bad cold. He asked whether there was an Adventist health center in the area, and was referred to Paradise Valley Sanitarium in National City. Again he was impressed with the spirit of service the staff provided. He especially admired the kindness of a student nurse who cared for an old man with Parkinson's disease.

Bookkeeping at Paradise Valley was done by hand in 1928, and the patients' journal was balanced at the end of each week. One week the clerk found a 45-cent overcharge in Porter's account. Credit manager Harley Rice immediately mailed a refund check with an apology. Porter promptly returned the check, claiming it was he who was indebted to the sanitarium staff.

A couple of months later, Porter inquired about the possibility of building a facility in Denver similar to the ones in California. He was directed to church officials, and as a result, he and his daughter, Dora

Porter Mason, gave $330,000 to build the Porter Sanitarium and Hospital on 40 acres that had been part of the original Porter family estate. At that time it was the largest single gift ever received by the Adventist church. An additional $50,000 gift was used to build a nurses' dormitory called Dora Porter Mason Hall, which today houses some of the hospital offices.

Attention to Details

Porter's interest in the hospital was clearly evident in his detailed suggestions to church leaders. He made a pencil sketch of the design he envisioned, including landscaping, dormitory, artesian well, an 11-acre pasture and 20 acres to be planted in corn and alfalfa. He even specified a fence built of "Colorado Special Wire."

Ground was broken in February 1929, with the earth so frozen that a fire was built to thaw a place for groundbreaking participants to dig their shovels. One year later between 4,000 and 5,000 guests attended the grand opening of the 80-bed hospital on February 16, 1930. Unfortunately, Mr. Porter was sick with the flu and unable to attend.

Starting a hospital at the beginning of the Great Depression brought many challenges, and Porter's early years were understandably difficult. Many patients could not pay their bills. Sometimes physicians with financial difficulties of their own, helped pay patients' bills. Employee salaries were reduced at least three times. In 1936 nurses received 35 cents an hour for special duty and 32 cents an hour for floor duty.

True to Its Purpose

"Our great burden is not that this new institution shall be a great, outstanding financial success, but rather that it shall find its place in the purpose of God and become the blessing in its community that its altruistic donors have purposed."—CHARLES RICE

While the Adventists assured Porter they would run the hospital debt-free, he was sympathetic to the financial difficulties of those early years. He had a room at the hospital where he occasionally stayed for hydrotherapy treatments. However, without regard for his generosity in establishing the hospital, he paid for these services as though he were a stranger.

Callboy's Work is Never Done

Delos Reeder, retired electrician, came to the Porter San at the end of 1941 and got a job as a callboy, receiving 27 cents an hour.

"We did a lot of work then that is not done by anybody now because at that time oxygen was not piped to the patient rooms. We had the old 100-pound tanks that I used to take to the rooms. I'd get the portable oxygen tent out of storage, and then fill the canister with ice. After I got everything plugged in and running, a nurse came in and set the amount of oxygen."

When they weren't doing anything else, the callboys stood at the front door to welcome guests and visitors. This also meant assisting sanitarium patients who came with trunks and suitcases containing the personal items needed for a lengthy stay.

"We had to move all their stuff into the rooms—private rooms with rugs on the floor," Reeder recalls. "We were more or less bellhops to them when they needed help. They just lived there for months."

Reeder also recalls that Porter had a severe shortage of employee housing during World War II. Some workers lived in the hospital and several single women lived in the nurses' dormitory. This situation changed after the war when "The Courts" apartments were built from recycled military barracks, which Reeder helped move from the Fort Carson U.S. Army base in Colorado Springs. For nearly 30 years The Courts housed employees and interns, as well as offices.

One of the hospital's notable leaders was Harley Rice, the son of Porter's second business manager Charles Rice. Young Harley had been the person at Paradise Valley Sanitarium who sent Henry Porter the 45-cent refund in 1928.

It's me, Lord

When his office telephone rang, Harley Rice always answered, "Rice speaking." Perhaps not even he realized how much of a habit this had become until one Sabbath morning during church service when he offered prayer. Members of the congregation knelt, bowed their heads and closed their eyes. In the silence of the moment, the hospital business manager began to pray.

"Rice speaking," he said.

While those attending church that morning may not remember the rest of his prayer, no one was in doubt as to who offered it, not even the Lord. —DR. JOHN DAVIS

Long-time employees, physicians and volunteers agree that the people at Porter Sanitarium and Hospital were like a big family. They remember picnics and ballgames on the front lawn, packing fruit baskets for employees at Christmastime, making fruitcakes for special friends of the hospital, and helping each other during snowstorms.

Memories of Long-time Employees

Two members of the Porter hospital family are sisters Lila Fehrer and Irene Howe. Now retired, the women live only a mile from the hospital and continue to serve as volunteers. Both joined the hospital in 1958. Fehrer was secretary to the administrator for 25 years, and Howe retired in 1988 with 30 years of service. Although at the beginning her medical terminology was limited to "appendectomy" and "tonsillectomy," Howe started as a medical transcriptionist. With the help of a medical dictionary and the kindness of her co-workers, her vocabulary quickly increased.

"I'd just say, 'I don't understand this at all,' and one of the others would come over and help me."

In addition, she observed a couple of autopsies.

"I thought, 'Oh, I don't know how I can handle this,' she says. "I just had to disassociate myself and think of it as a learning experience."

Post World War II brought some unusual challenges to the Porter medical staff, which was not open to adding many new physicians. As a consequence, a group of doctors converted a tuberculosis sanatorium into a general hospital that became Swedish Medical Center. The resulting competition between the hospitals was partially resolved with the creation of a combined medical staff.

Under this arrangement, physicians on the staff of one hospital automatically had privileges at the other, explains John Davis, who was on the staff from 1952 until he retired in 1985. While ownership of each hospital remained unchanged, the combined staff reduced duplication of medical staff business. Additionally, the hospitals agreed not to duplicate certain services. For example, Swedish developed a strong emergency department, while Porter focused on obstetrics and pediatrics. During 18 years as administrator from 1959–1977, Olof Moline helped develop this plan which strengthened the Porter medical staff.

Over time the hospital grew, adding to the physical plant and increasing the number of patient beds. When Porter's son, William E. Porter, died in 1959, he bequeathed to the hospital a residual portion of the estate, which amounted to a million dollars. This helped fund a $2.5 million addition. Subsequent building programs eventually brought the total patient beds to 369.

With the medical staff pretty well developed, the arrival of Ron Sackett as administrator in 1978 brought a new focus on services and programs, and the relationship with Swedish eventually dissolved.

Today's Porter Adventist Hospital is known for its cardiovascular services, transplant program, state-of-the-art cancer center and women's center for minimally invasive surgery. Additionally, Porter's success made it possible to build a sister hospital in Littleton, and to support construction of Avista Adventist Hospital in Louisville to replace Boulder Memorial Hospital, which was sold in 1989.

Littleton Adventist Hospital came about when Porter officials learned that a California developer had purchased property south of Denver. They bought about 40 acres in the area and opened an 85-bed facility in 1989. It has grown to 139 beds and is now building a $40 million expansion to meet the needs of a rapidly growing market.

The Adventist hospitals in Colorado today stand as memorials to a Denver businessman with a generous heart, and they bear testimony to an unidentified therapist who turned down a one-dollar tip, a student nurse who compassionately cared for her elderly patient, and a conscientious bookkeeper who returned a 45-cent overpayment, as well as many others whose Christian service exemplifies the healing ministry of Christ.

SOURCES

Rymes, Marion, *Porter Memorial Hospital: Its Birth and Life*, Denver, Colorado: Porter Memorial Hospital, 1978.

Robinson, Dores Eugene, *The Story of Our Health Message*, Nashville, Tennessee: Southern Publishing Association. 1943.

"Sixty Years of Caring," Denver, Colorado: Porter Memorial Hospital, 1990.

Interviews: Dr. John Davis, Lila Fehrer, Irene Howe, Delos Reeder and Ron Sackett.

Part 2

Overseas Growth

Chapter 19

Diamond Mines, Dispensaries and Dedication

Pioneers in Foreign Lands

When the early Adventist missionaries sailed to Africa, the South Seas, South America and Asia, they expected to face all sorts of diseases and living conditions, as well as strange languages, cultures, superstitions and even hostilities. But how could they have imagined that a century later their church would operate more than 100 overseas hospitals, plus dozens of clinics and dispensaries in virtually every corner of the earth?

From the jungles of the Amazon to the deserts of Africa and the streets of Hong Kong and Sydney, the Seventh-day Adventist Church has served the healthcare needs of people around the world for more than a century. The church began sending missionaries outside the United States in the late 1800s, but the most dramatic growth in the overseas medical work occurred after 1915. By this time, the early sanitariums in the United States were involved in strengthening their programs, while the new Adventist medical school in California had begun producing qualified physicians prepared to expand the church's healthcare outreach overseas.

The first overseas medical missionaries came from Battle Creek. These were pioneers in every sense. Many braved regions where no other Americans or Europeans had ever gone. After long and often rough sea voyages, they traveled for days by horse, mule cart, bicycle or on foot to reach their assigned posts. They encountered bandits, disease, suspicion, superstition, primitive living conditions and political uprisings. Mission life was filled with hardships and challenges, as well as rewards and blessings.

While many early missionaries were doctors and nurses, all missionaries had some medical training. Initially, this was to equip them to care for themselves and their families, but finding sickness and disease wherever they went, they sought to relieve human suffering in any way they could.

This explains why some of the early healthcare stories from overseas come from missionary teachers and ministers. For example, Eric Hare, famous Adventist storyteller, was a teacher and school principal in Burma (now Myanmar), but he was also a trained nurse. Christopher Robinson, founder of the Malawi Mission in Africa, was another trained nurse. Orley and Lillian Ford served in South America with only four months' training in medical techniques.

Sometimes a missionary minister or teacher married a nurse who carried the healthcare responsibilities of a mission or school. In fact, some of today's hospitals began as home dispensaries operated by these women. Of course, a number of husband-wife physician teams made significant contributions to the development of Adventist mission hospitals. Most of the treatment rooms and dispensaries operated by the early missionaries did not develop into permanent facilities.

The historical backgrounds and stories in the following pages are organized by continents, with the exception of Central America and the Caribbean, which are included in the section called Inter-American. No conscious effort was made to balance the space devoted to each region, although the resulting imbalance may somewhat reflect the actual development of facilities in each area. As a rule, in areas where there were more missionaries, there were more hospitals, and thus more stories and resources are available. Nevertheless, the stories in this section help illustrate the beginnings of Adventist healthcare outside the United States and Canada.

Chapter 20

AFRICA—Diamonds in the Rough

Complicated Delivery

"Once I rode in the big Kanya [Kanye] *hospital truck, with its huge tires for travel in the desert; mostly we ploughed through sand in second or low gear. We went to visit our far-flung Kalahari clinics. In addition to medicines, food, bedding, and diesel fuel for the truck, we carried 42 passengers! We were out for over two weeks. It was July, winter in the Southern Hemisphere, and cold at night.... One evening we arrived at the farthest clinic. Our nurses there were happy to see us. They had a woman in labor for four days who was unable to deliver. I was to do a Cesarean delivery, but the major surgery pack containing everything necessary had been autoclaved (sterilized) so many times that the sutures had gelled! What to do?*

"I asked the nurses to boil common thread and attempted a procedure I had read about but had never before tried to do. This was to do a partial symphysiotomy (surgical separation of the symphysis pubis). It was now night, and the only light available was a kerosene lantern with a dirty smoked glass chimney! I made the incision, and, with our assistants, delivered a yelling baby boy with a lot of meconium in the waters, indicating fetal distress. We delivered the placenta, sutured the incision, cleaned up the baby, and went on our way early the next morning. In three days when we came back, mother and baby were fine!" —DR. DUNBAR SMITH

The discovery of diamonds on the farm of a generous Seventh-day Adventist family in South Africa led to the earliest Adventist healthcare ventures in Africa. Members of the Wessels family visited church headquarters in Michigan several times, and some attended Battle Creek College. Over time they assisted in developing a number of Adventist schools and hospitals in Africa and other parts of the world.

In their homeland of South Africa, the Wessels family built the Claremont Sanitarium in 1897. Two familiar names connected with that facility were Nellie Druillard, a key figure in the histories of Tennessee Christian Medical Center and Riverside Hospital in Nashville, and Dr. Kate Lindsay, Adventist pioneer in nursing education. The South African government took over the Claremont San during the Anglo-Boer War in the early 1900s. After the war the Wessels operated it again until it burned in 1905.

The family also donated a former orphanage to establish the Cape Sanitarium in South Africa, which operated from 1904 until the 1930s. Many graduates of the Cape San's school of nursing helped establish other healthcare facilities in Africa.

Adventists from the United States and Europe began arriving in the late 1800s and early 1900s to pioneer missions, schools and healthcare facilities on the continent. Among these was George James, a Battle Creek College graduate with a burden for the indigenous people of Africa. When he learned that the church's Foreign Mission Board had no funds for this work in 1893, he sold everything he owned except his violin, and went to Malawi as a self-supporting missionary. He preached the gospel, played his violin and treated the sick using methods he had learned at Battle Creek, making him the first Adventist medical missionary to Africa's indigenous people.

One of the most significant Adventist pioneers in Africa was W.H. Anderson, who arrived in 1893 and worked in this part of the world for 50 years. He personally selected sites for many of the mission stations and healthcare facilities, some of which remain today.

Typically, an early African mission station consisted of a school, medical dispensary or clinic, and administrative offices. Missionaries usually filled multiple roles—teacher, nurse, preacher and administrator. Their facilities were primitive, and they treated hundreds of people under shade trees, in tents or mud-and-thatch huts. They saw patients on their verandas, mixed medicines in their bathrooms and did surgeries on kitchen tables.

Having few resources, limited equipment and untrained personnel, they treated all sorts of diseases ranging from malaria and dysentery to tuberculosis, leprosy, tropical ulcers and chiggers. Many had to deal with superstition and fear, as well as hippos, lions and other wild animals. Life was difficult and too many died or saw their co-workers and loved ones die in service to the people of Africa.

In 1902 the church purchased 50 acres for a mission station in Malawi. This station, called Malamulo, would become a major Adventist mission center with a school and hospital. Today's Malamulo Hospital, the oldest Adventist healthcare facility in Africa, likely started as a dispensary or clinic operated by nurses from Battle Creek and the Cape Sanitarium.

Handmade Bricks and More

Construction equipment, bricks and timber for the new hospital in Malawi were secured on the mission property or produced from materials on hand. Women carried water on their heads from a nearby stream for hydrotherapy treatments. Like everything else, even the patient beds were hand-built. With the last bed in place, the staff was ready for the first inpatients.

Christopher Robinson, a trained nurse from Cape Town, headed Malamulo from 1911 to 1919, and helped establish a strong mission program, including the first permanent hospital facility. Soon after the hospital opened, the wards were so full the staff had to remove the hand-built beds and place patients side-by-side on the floor. It is reported that Dr. Carl Birkenstock, the hospital's first medical director, and nurse Daisy Ingle cared for more than 17,000 patients in the first eight months of 1926.

Birkenstock, a South African, graduated from the College of Medical Evangelists (CME) in Loma Linda, California, and was former director of the Cape Sanitarium. Shortly after joining Malamulo in 1925, he established a program for sufferers of leprosy. He had 100 brick huts constructed in 1936 to house these patients.

Malamulo continued to grow over the years and now provides more than 200 patient beds. With improved methods for treating leprosy, patients no longer must live at the hospital. Instead, Malamulo is now a designated leprosy control center for the Lower Shire River Valley, and doctors travel to patients' villages to provide care.

Crushing Hospital Bills

Leaders at Malamulo during the 1970s devised a plan to help patients pay their bills and earn an income, while making it possible for the hospital to pave one of its main roads. No gravel was to be found any place in the area, but there were plenty of rocks. Medical director Dr. G.M. Burnham hired patients for the slow and laborious task of hammering the large rocks into gravel-size pieces. Part of what they earned was applied to their hospital bill and the rest was theirs. It took about two years to crush enough rock to build the road. —RAY PELTON, RETIRED ASSOCIATE DIRECTOR, HEALTH AND TEMPERANCE DEPARTMENT, GENERAL CONFERENCE OF SEVENTH-DAY ADVENTISTS

By the 1920s and 1930s an increasing number of CME graduates were coming to Africa to build permanent healthcare facilities. They were responsible for everything from making bricks to pulling teeth and delivering babies. If they didn't know how to roof a building or do a hernia operation, they learned on the job. They planted peanuts and citrus crops, operated leper colonies, and held mobile clinics under the wings of small aircraft. At times their hospitals were closed or taken over during wars or other times of trouble. In other instances, governments assisted in building mission hospitals.

For instance, when Ethiopia's Emperor Haile Selassie I was crowned in 1930, the Adventists' Scandinavian Union sent a congratulatory message. This gesture eventually resulted in his building the Empress Zauditu Memorial Adventist Hospital, which the church operated from 1932 to 1976, except for a brief time during World War II. In Nigeria, the leader of the Yoruba tribe gave 40 acres to build Ile-Ife Hospital in the 1940s. And, while the Sierra Leone government did not build a mission hospital, it turned over the Masanga Leprosy Hospital to the church in 1965.

The story is told that to find a proper site for a hospital in Africa, early missionaries traveled by train to the end of the line. They bought a team of oxen and went as far as the animals could take them. After that, they walked as far as they could walk. At that point someone declared, "This is the spot where the hospital will be."

Challenges of an Outpost Mission

"I knew when I married Kenneth that he wanted to go to the boonies, and Gimbie was about as 'boonie' as you could get," says Aileen Saunders, retired missionary who served with her husband in Pakistan and Ethiopia from 1957 to 1967.

The 300-mile trip from Addis Ababa to Gimbie Hospital meant driving over 200 miles of gravel road and 80 miles of washed-out ruts carved into the earth by large trucks hauling loads of coffee beans. With nearly 30 rivers to ford, and broken-down trucks frequently blocking the way, Saunders says it usually took about eight hours to drive the 80-mile stretch.

Although she declared her first ride on the Gimbie road would be her last, for the next five years she made three trips a year to Addis Ababa to buy food and supplies. With the biggest shopping trip scheduled for January, she would hire coffee trucks to haul her purchases to Gimbie.

"Then I would go again in April, just before the rainy season to pick up anything I wasn't able to get in January. In November I'd get what we needed to last until the big trip in January," she explains.

As the unofficial purchasing director, she managed to get everything the hospital and missionaries needed in Addis Ababa.

"The government medicine store carried a lot of stuff and there were several other medical companies. By searching around I could usually get what we needed."

Like all missionaries, Saunders looked forward to receiving mail. Because Gimbie did not have mail service, the hospital sent a runner to the nearest postal delivery station every other week. He walked three days, picked up the mail, and walked another three days back to the hospital. Saunders says when the mail came everything else stopped.

Serving in a mission outpost like Gimbie is fraught with risk and danger, a fact that did not escape the Saunders family. Tragically, their youngest child died of unexplainable causes at Gimbie.

In spite of their loss, Saunders says her family loved it there. She believes her husband's happiest years were at the Gimbie Hospital. In five years, he took only three weeks of vacation.

"He used to say that in the United States, there was always another doctor. If you weren't there, another doctor was within a few miles. But at Gimbie there wasn't another doctor for 100 miles."

Today Adventists operate between 20 and 25 hospitals, and dozens of dispensaries on the continent of Africa. For more than a century, hundreds of missionary doctors and nurses have served here, each with his or her unique experiences. Following are stories shared by two families who pioneered medical work in Angola and Uganda.

SOURCES

Cripps, Jean, "Early Days at Malamulo Mission," *Review and Herald*, May 16, 1957.

Schaffner, Marlowe H., M.D., "At Work Among the Lepers at Songa Mission Hospital," *The Medical Evangelist*, August 1955.

Smith, Dunbar W., M.D., *The Travels, Triumphs and Vicissitudes of Dunbar W. Smith, M.D.*, Loma Linda, California: Dunbar W. Smith, M.D. 1994.

Wagner, William, M.D., "Ile-Ife Mission Hospital School of Nursing," SDA Document File 3541.30, Loma Linda University, Heritage Room.

Wagner, William, M.D., "To Improve Food Supply for Masanga Leprosarium, *LLU Alumni Journal*, July-August 1969.

Interviews: Ray Pelton and Aileen Saunders.

Chapter 21

AFRICA—The Parsons in Angola

Life and Death Matters

"Will I get well?" the African wanted to know.

Dr. Roy Parsons dared not make that promise. He had only recently arrived at the Bongo Mission Hospital and needed to gain the Africans' confidence. Speaking through an interpreter, he chose his words carefully, explaining that he thought the man would recover, but could not guarantee it.

The man, who seemed much older than his 60 years, turned to the villagers accompanying him and started talking. The doctor could not understand a word of their long conversation.

"If he is not operated, will he die?" the interpreter finally asked.

"Yes. He has no hope of recovering without the operation" the doctor replied.

Again the old man conferred with his companions. After a few minutes he sat upright and signaled his interpreter to tell the doctor his decision.

"If he dies, it will be without a gash."

The Parsons family called Bongo Mission Hospital home for more than 43 years. After graduating from the College of Medical Evangelists in 1929 and studying tropical medicine in Portugal, Parsons—with his wife, Mabel, three-year-old Roy, Jr., and baby David—arrived at the Angola hospital December 1, 1931. In the following years they experienced the many challenges and rewards, as well as heartaches and sacrifices of overseas service.

Adventists originally came to Angola in 1924 and established a mission station in the Lepi region, 200 miles inland at a mile-high elevation. The mission director's wife operated a small dispensary until Dr. A.N. Tonge arrived in 1926 to direct the medical work and establish what later became Bongo Mission Hospital. While supervising construction of the hospital, the doctor held clinics on a veranda and used his bathroom as a dispensary. He left Bongo shortly after Parsons arrived.

By this time the mission consisted of four small buildings clustered at the base of a mountain. Mrs. Parsons wrote letters home describing their humble working conditions.

No Conveniences of Home

"*In this operating room there was a folding field operating room table that had cost the hospital $75, a Harvest Ingathering donation.* (An annual solicitation of funds for the church's humanitarian activities. Now simply called "Ingathering.") *Its cost had been deducted from the first year's operating budget of $600.... The surgical instruments consisted of an army field operating kit.... At least we could take care of emergency wounds and do amputations.*

"*The two wards comprising the hospital had no beds. There were a few ticks filled with grass that could serve as beds—on the floor....*

"*The dispensary...consisted of one large room and two smaller ones. One of the small rooms served as a supply room, the other as an examining room. The larger room was the utility room where the ironing was done, the fomentations given, the syringes boiled, and later on when surgery was done, it was in that room....*

"*Kerosene boxes served as seats for those taking treatments with fomentations. The fomentation tank was a kerosene tin, with a rack on the bottom to keep the cloths from getting wet....*

"*The porch across the back of the dispensary was used for treating...tropical ulcers, and for dental extractions. A square, homemade table on the porch served as a place for the bottles of medicine, and medicine cups, the rags and bandages made from old sheets, contributed by the missionaries, and the homemade medicine for the leg ulcers....*

"*The patient always came accompanied. The women would come with a wide cone-shaped basket with a hoe. The men would come carrying a small homemade axe. There would be someone in the group with a bow and arrows, and once in a while, a spear.... There might be a live chicken and some corn meal. A few of the people might bring beans tied up in a piece of cloth, or a ball of dried black-eyed pea leaves. There might be a blanket to sleep in at night, or a mat to spread on the ground as a bed mattress. Others...cut grass to sleep on....*

"*The 'sick village'...was made up of...wigwam-like pole and grass structures large enough for a person to lie down...with a fire burning in the middle for warmth.... The ground around these temporary houses was cluttered with corn cobs, corn husks, chicken feathers, rope bark strips, twigs...ashes from the fires, bits of sugar cane stocks or corn stocks.*

Water for drinking was contained in homemade clay pots.... The odor of human excreta was strong....

"*Bathing was done in a little stream.... The sicker the patient, the less frequent the bathing. The debilitated sat around their fires...with meager clothing....*

"*It was apparent that the sick village must be moved. Sanitary conditions had to be established. The yards...[needed to be] swept up, with the refuse discarded far away in a compost pile.*

"*There were dispensary patients [with] sores and tropical ulcers, malaria, dental caries...and conjunctivitis.... Many needed hospitalization.... But there were no beds. There was no furniture. Just space. There was a big job to be done, and right away.*"

The hospital was extremely isolated, lacking such modern conveniences as running water and electricity. Water had to be carried three miles to the mission. With no grocery stores in the region, Parsons developed a dairy and farm to raise food for patients and his family, which increased by two with the births of another son and a daughter. Later he kept wild animals such as deer and impala on the hospital grounds for patients to enjoy.

Most of the time, Parsons was the only physician at Bongo. European and American nurses worked with him and operated a school of nursing. The doctor's days began before dawn and continued into the night with an overcrowded schedule of patient visits and surgeries. Periodically he treated patients and performed surgeries at outlying clinics. Regardless of ability to pay, he never turned anyone away.

Bongo-style Surgery Suite

"*Until the storage room was converted into an operating room, we did surgery in the same room where we treated tropical ulcers. The oversized table in the operating room was also used for patient examinations...and for spreading the fomentation cloths for drying. The sterile drapes could not cover the table because of its width. It really was a problem for two tall men to meet in the middle to do their work. Someone had to hold the patient's hands during surgery. The secretary-treasurer of the Angola Union assisted and sometimes gave ether. I did the circulating, keeping the water hot on the wood-burning stove that was in the same room!*"

A share of what Parsons learned of surgery, he learned on the job—with a copy of *Gray's Anatomy* handy for reference if needed during a procedure. Herniotomies were most common, but it would take experience for the missionary doctor to consider them routine. He used to say he sometimes felt like the old general practitioner, who when asked how to do a herniotomy, replied, "Cut the skin, and the superficial fascia, and then proceed cautiously."

One of Parsons' first hernia surgeries took more than two hours. It was a normal sized hernia and didn't appear to be complicated. After studying *Gray's Anatomy*, he proceeded, only to discover that the actual location of vessels and nerves in the human anatomy varies from the standard book drawings, depending on the patient's size. Also inflammation and pathology distort internal structures, making identification difficult for the inexperienced eye. All of this was complicated by the fact that ether used to keep the patient asleep, volatizes rapidly at high altitudes.

"Experience would be gained later," Mrs. Parsons wrote. "Speed would come with practice."

Life in Angola was not easy for the Parsons. Their letters speak of lack of equipment and instruments, adverse working conditions, professional isolation and the doctor's desire for access to a good library. Discouragement came easy. Yet the Parsons saw a need, they felt called of God to this mission, and gave it their best—committed to whatever challenges each new day brought their way.

"Our diseases run by seasons," the doctor wrote. Malaria was most severe from May to August, and lobar pneumonia from April to July. Eye diseases, tropical ulcers, tuberculosis and leprosy were common all year long. People had confidence in Parsons and came to him with all sorts of illnesses and injuries.

Innovative Ambulance Service

"Patients sometimes arrived via 'tipoy,' a hammock-like mode of transportation made by slinging two gunny sacks that had been sown [sic] together with bark rope and suspended from a long pole carried on the shoulders of two men. To prevent the sack from folding over the patient, the two corners at the top were tied to a cross stick with bark rope. The bottom was gathered up and knotted, then tied to the long pole. The patient clung to the long pole for support, while being swung and jostled all the way to the mission hospital. The larger the number of people accompanying the patient, the higher his or her status in the village. Women accompanied maternity cases."

෭

The Parsons made their home at Bongo Mission Hospital until 1975. This is where they raised their family, and this is where two sons, David and Robert, returned to serve as a physician and medical technologist respectively. When his father officially retired in 1968, David became medical director and his wife, Leona, was director of nurses.

Planning to continue the family tradition at Bongo, David and Leona built a home, furnished it with appliances from the United States, and brought AAA Guernsey cows for the dairy. However, a 1975 political uprising forced them out of the country. Drs. Roy and David stayed until the last possible minute. Then early one morning they slipped out, boarded a plane parked about a mile from the hospital, and leaving all their earthly belongings behind, escaped in the midst of gunfire.

SOURCES

"Dr. Roy Parsons, Medical Missionary In Angola," *LLU Alumni Journal*, January 1963.

"Missionaries Flee from the Congo When Endangered by Fierce Tribal Fighting," *LLU Alumni Journal*, July-August 1963.

Unpublished manuscripts and letters supplied by the Parsons family.

Chapter 22

AFRICA—Mission to Uganda

Calls in the Night

Many times there was a tap on the door, or a lantern at our bedroom window as a worker called us to the hospital in the night. Someone has fallen from a bicycle. A buffalo has gored a villager. A woman has been in labor for four days. A child with a high fever is having convulsions. A lion chased a man up a tree and has eaten most of the flesh from his feet. A boy has fallen from a truck and broken his leg. A woman has been struck by lightning. A man was pierced in the stomach with a spear. So goes the night. Tomorrow is another day. —DR. MILDRED STILSON

As the ship called *Llandovery Castle* docked at Mombasa, Kenya, in January 1949, young Drs. Donald and Mildred Stilson looked forward to being medical missionaries in Africa. After gaining additional experience in surgery and obstetrics, the 1946 graduates of the College of Medical Evangelists were excited about their assignment to a new hospital in Uganda. They had another reason to be excited, too, for they were expecting their first child. Having suffered from both morning sickness and seasickness on the long voyage from England to East Africa, Dr. Mildred was happy to be on land again.

Sixteen months earlier the Stilsons had packed their worldly goods—plus items they would need for mission life in Africa—and left them in New York City while they went to London to study tropical medicine and take the qualifying examinations to practice in a British country.

Finally they were on the African continent, with no idea how long they must wait for their crates and trunks. As children of missionaries themselves, both knew the wait could be several months. So it was no small miracle when they discovered that the freighter containing their shipment—including a 1944 Studebaker and a small collapsible trailer—was also docked in Mombassa, bow-to-bow with the *Llandovery Castle*.

In a short time they had packed their car and trailer and begun the 1,000-mile journey inland to Kendu Mission Hospital in Kenya, where Dr. Donald Abbott would orient them to medical care in Africa. They must learn how to run a mission dispensary and gain some experience in complicated surgeries and deliveries under circumstances far different from what they were used to. Abbott put them to work immediately. Unfortunately, the first whiff of tropical ulcers, infected injuries and other unfamiliar smells of the mission hospital sent Dr. Mildred straight out the back door where she says she vomited "everything from the boots up!"

First chance he had, Dr. Donald traveled 500 miles to Uganda to see the new hospital at Ishaka, where he and his wife would serve. He took the overnight steamer across northern Lake Victoria, and then traveled by car another 250 miles. Located practically on the equator and a mile above sea level, the hospital property was set on a hill at the junction of three main roads, one coming from the capital city of Kampala, another going south to Rwanda and the third leading northwest to the Belgian Congo. From the top of the hill he could see the Volcanic Mountains, home of the famous gorilla sanctuary. The new mission hospital would be the closest healthcare facility for nearly a quarter of a million people living in this region.

"What a privilege to serve God in such a beautiful place," he thought.

Expecting to find a hospital structure at least partially completed, he was surprised to find only one corner of foundation measuring about two feet on each side. From his first visit to Ishaka, Stilson discovered his work involved many skills he had not learned in medical school. In Uganda he supervised brick-making, plumbing, septic tank construction, roofing, furniture and cabinet design and construction, as well as installation of a steam autoclave, portable X-ray unit and dark room—just to name a few of his responsibilities. Every bit of concrete and plaster was prepared at the building site, and then carried in flat basins on workmen's heads.

Unable to wait until the hospital was completed, the Stilsons temporarily moved into the first building in February 1950. It was a brick structure with corrugated iron roof and would eventually serve as the missionary nurses' residence. In no time patients began coming. Given no other choice, the doctors held clinic on their back porch and mixed medicines in their kitchen until they could move into the hospital.

While Dr. Donald oversaw construction, Dr. Mildred ran the pharmacy, kept the accounts and supervised the sewing of sheets, gowns and operating room linens.

After about six months, a Danish nurse transferred to Ishaka from Kendu Mission Hospital. Else Brandt was the first of several nurses from Europe, Australia, the West Indies and North America who served at Ishaka Adventist Hospital over the years. These women trained young Africans to assist as ward nurses and "dressers," or aides. Those who were midwives assisted with routine deliveries, and otherwise provided valuable assistance to doctors and patients.

By the end of 1950, the hospital was sufficiently completed to accommodate a few inpatients. Dr. Donald and D.K. Short, a pastor who stayed at Ishaka for several months, personally built 80 beds to furnish the wards.

"We had brought some woodworking tools from the States," Stilson explains. "I took ordinary flat iron springs such as you'd find on a cot, and bolted them to the wooden head and foot pieces which we had made. Then we put a coconut fiber mat on the springs, and that is where the patients slept."

"The Lord surely walked with us on our ward rounds and guided in the care of patients who constantly increased in number, coming in all weather, on foot, by bus, by bicycle or on crude litters carried by relatives," says Dr. Mildred. Diseases and injuries ran the gamut—from bicycle accidents to hippo attacks, emergency surgeries, complicated obstetrics, tuberculosis, sleeping sickness, malaria and "a whole array of tropical parasites."

Members of the large population of East Indians living in Uganda during the 1950s raised funds to build a separate Asian ward at Ishaka. In separating the Africans and Asians, the ward also separated the Moslems and Hindus. Having spent her childhood in India, Dr. Mildred understood the Hindu customs, class distinctions and some of their language. So she naturally assumed responsibility for most of the Indian patients.

Challenge of the Ages

Both Asian and African women appreciated a woman doctor caring for them. Dr. Mildred always looked for opportunities to help improve their lifestyle and health. Too often her well-intended counsel went unheeded, but one patient raised her hopes that she might make a lasting difference in at least one family. The woman was a Mukima married to a local chief, a privileged man who had attended Oxford University. She was extremely obese and suffered high blood pressure when she came to the doctor.

"I talked with her about diet, exercise, habits and so forth. She and her husband asked intelligent questions and we discussed things thoroughly," the doctor recalls.

On the day the woman was discharged, her blood pressure was under control, and she and her husband seemed interested in changing their lifestyle.

"Thank you so very much, 'Doctoress,' for what you have done for my wife, and the time you have spent with us," the husband said.

They seemed so pleased with the care and attention they'd received that Dr. Mildred did not anticipate the husband's parting comment.

"But you know, we can't do the things you taught us."

The doctor's face must have shown a combination of surprise, puzzlement and disappointment. The man standing before her looked almost helpless as he explained, "Our fathers didn't do these things."

Another mother's story further illustrates some of the challenges of medical missionary work in Uganda at that time. The woman delivered quadruplets, which in most cultures would be cause for celebration. In fact, Uganda's British protectorate government gave a "Queen's Bounty" to parents of multiple birth children to help feed and clothe the extra babies. But for the African woman, a multiple birth was a sign of bad luck, and this mother would have nothing to do with her babies. The Ishaka doctors and nurses cared for them until time came for the mother to leave the hospital. She grudgingly took her babies home. Unfortunately, the hospital staff later learned that all four died of starvation.

Today the Stilsons hope things have changed in Uganda, yet they know it takes several generations to change deep-seated cultural traditions. Also, some of the changes initiated by missionaries to improve the lives of those they serve actually create other problems. For example, many African women suffered from rickets as a result of poor nutrition. After missionaries taught them to improve their diet, they began having larger babies—and complicated deliveries.

Not all the stories from Ishaka Adventist Hospital ended on a sad note, of course. One of the patients was an achondroplastic dwarf. While her body proportions were fairly normal, she had extremely short arms and legs, typical of this condition. When she became pregnant, it was determined that she would require a Caesarian section. The doctor foresaw no problem, but the expectant mother was convinced that she would not live through the ordeal. Just before surgery, she had one request.

"Please let me see my baby before I die?"

Although the doctor tried to calm her fears, the woman was not convinced until after she delivered and held her baby in her arms. Both mother and baby did fine.

Family Matters

Five-year-old Enid stood at the head of the operating table wearing a surgical mask and holding a bottle of ether.

"Listen carefully to Mommy," Dr. Mildred told her obedient helper.

Drip, drip, drip. Little Enid didn't miss a beat as she carefully followed her mother's instructions. Watching a surgery was nothing new for the child, who had often played in the operating room while her parents worked on a patient, but this was the first time she had helped.

Her daddy was in Kampala when the patient came to the mission hospital in need of emergency minor surgery, and the overworked nurses were all busy. Dr. Mildred knew her little girl could handle the job.

In addition to running the mission hospital, the Stilsons had a family to care for. Eric was born at Ishaka in 1953. With two children at home, plus a hospital full of patients, the doctors never had much spare time. When the children reached school age, they took lessons by correspondence.

"I tried to be at home mornings until clinic consultation time," she says "This worked well unless I had to help with major surgery. When both Dr. Donald and I had to be at the hospital for extended periods, we took Enid and Eric with us. They could nap, read, color and play in the one private room. If the private room happened to be occupied, we put masks on the kids and they sat quietly in the corner of the surgery. They had lots of pets and nice play places in the garden around our house."

After 11 years of service, the Stilsons left Ishaka in 1961. By then the campus consisted of the main hospital, an outpatient dispensary, a church (which also served as a school), utility buildings for laundry, sewing, carpentry and the electric light generator, and houses for the African staff and expatriate doctors and nurses. In recent years physicians from the Philippines and Africa have served in the medical-director post at Ishaka Adventist Hospital.

SOURCES

"Ankole Mission Hospital in Remote Uganda is Growing Project," *LLU Alumni Journal*, September 1960.

Interviews and Notes: Drs. Donald and Mildred Stilson.

Chapter 23

ASIA—Blessings, Bombs and Tiger Tales

Unknown Soldiers

The story is told that during an anti-American uprising in the 1960s, an angry mob filled the eight-lane road in front of Karachi Adventist Hospital. Built in 1951, the hospital was the outgrowth of a clinic started in Pakistan in 1947, and was sometimes called the American Hospital

On this occasion, protesters stomped on American flags and even burned the American library across the street. Later someone told hospital leaders that had it not been for the soldiers stationed on the wall around the compound, the hospital would have been burned, too.

"What soldiers?" the hospital leaders asked.

Listening to reports of eyewitnesses, they realized it was only by a miracle that the Karachi Adventist Hospital had been saved.

The countries of Asia began attracting Adventist missionaries as early as the 1890s, when doctors and nurses arrived in Calcutta, India. By the early 1900s, others were responding to the needs of this vast continent. Dr. S.A. Lockwood and a group of Japanese physicians opened a sanitarium in Kobe, Japan, in 1903. In the same year, Drs. Harry and Maude Miller, Drs. Arthur and Bertha Selmon and two nurses went to China. Dr. Ollie Oberholtzer began working in Burma (Myanmar) in 1907. Dr. Riley Russell arrived in Korea in 1908. Also about this time, Australian missionaries were operating health retreats in Indonesia.

Hundreds of missionaries went to China, Southern Asia and the Far East—working in rented storefronts or dispensaries at mission homes, offices and schools. It was not unusual for them to care for patients the same day they reached their posts of duty. In fact, in Soonan, Korea, Russell found people waiting for him at the train station when he arrived.

In most Asian countries, government officials welcomed the missionaries and many times provided land, money and/or influence to build hospitals. For example, China's "Young Marshall," and nationalist leader Chiang Kai-shek gave money for sanitariums in that country; a zamindar in India gave land and money to build Giffard Memorial

Hospital; and President Syngman Rhee intervened to help Seoul Adventist Hospital purchase land after the Korean War.

Asia was a continent for the hardy and adventuresome. Missionaries Herbert and Thelma Smith were among those who made the long journey into west China in the late 1920s. Traveling 1,500 miles from Shanghai through the rapids and gorges of the Yangtze River, they stopped long enough for Thelma to deliver their first child. Unfortunately, Herbert was murdered less than two years after arriving in China. Thelma remained in mission work, devoting her life to the people of China and Taiwan.

Dr. Theodore Flaiz, director of the church's medical work from 1946 to 1966, wrote about some of his hunting experiences while he was a young missionary in India. Both he and his sharpshooter wife saved several farmers' cattle from tigers, leopards and other wild animals. As a foreigner, Flaiz was among the few who could own a gun in India and thus was permitted to kill wild animals that threatened cattle or crops.

Wars played a significant part in the history of Adventist healthcare in Asia, notably the Japanese and communist invasions of China, World Wars I and II, the Korean War and the Vietnam War. Some hospitals closed temporarily, but others never reopened. Some suffered severe damage. Some were occupied for a time and then returned to the church. When the Japanese vacated the Manila Sanitarium after World War II, they detonated a bomb in the middle of the hospital, causing heavy damage. In contrast, when they occupied the Adventist hospital in Penang, Malaysia, they added a wing—which is still called the Japanese Wing.

While war disrupted or closed some medical work, it also provided the means to build or equip hospitals. Some facilities received free equipment and building supplies from the United Nations following World War II. The Pusan Hospital in Korea was built at the request of South Korea President Rhee following the Korean War. In Vietnam, Saigon Adventist Hospital had use of a fully furnished United States Army hospital from 1973 to 1975.

In spite of less than ideal circumstances, Adventist healthcare developed more rapidly in Asia than any other part of the world except North America. Unfortunately, most of the hospitals established in Asia between 1900 and 1945 no longer exist. Of the 40 or so remaining in 2000, only eight were begun before World War II. The oldest is Simla Sanitarium and Hospital in India, established by Dr. Herman Menkel in 1915. Today's Penang Adventist Hospital came into being when Dr. J.E. Gardner moved to Malaysia in 1925—after being denied permission to work in Indonesia. That was the same year Flaiz negotiated an agreement to build Giffard Memorial Hospital in India.

Both the Manila Sanitarium and Hospital and Tokyo Adventist Hospital opened in 1928. Dr. Horace Hall started the Manila facility with a dispensary and 10-bed hospital set up in a couple of mission houses. In Japan, a handful of church members raised most of the money for a 20-bed hospital in Tokyo, with labor provided by students and faculty of Japan Junior College and the Japan Union Mission staff.

Important growth continued throughout the 1930s. Dr. George Rue moved to Seoul and opened a clinic in an old pottery factory. Dr. George A. Nelson started another clinic that soon outgrew itself in Surat, India. In Bangkok Dr. Ralph Waddell began treating patients in rented shop houses. Each of these efforts has grown and continues to serve thousands of patients every year.

The second half of the 20th century saw other hospitals begun in Okinawa, Korea, Taiwan, Vietnam, Singapore, Indonesia, the Philippines, Pakistan, India, Nepal, Sri Lanka and Hong Kong. While some of these operated only a few years, new medical endeavors continued throughout the century. Today India and the Philippines lead in the number of Adventist hospitals in Asia, with approximately 10 each.

SOURCES

Flaiz, Theodore R. M.D., *Moonlit Trails in Indian Jungles*, Washington, D.C.: Review and Herald Publishing Association, 1938.

Ogle, Mary S., *In Spite of Danger*, Washington, D.C.: Review and Herald Publishing Association, 1969.

Interview: Aileen Saunders.

Chapter 24

ASIA—For the Love of China

Wartime Rescue

Riding in the back of an ambulance after the 1938 bombing of Hankow, Dr. Harry Miller saw that a small dispensary had been hit. When he stopped to see if anybody had been hurt, he heard a cry coming from underneath the pile of debris. He began digging through the concrete rubble until his hands bled. Finally he found a clinic worker with a baby in his arms. Miller reached out to free them and carried the child to safety.

From the time Adventist doctors and nurses arrived in the early 1900s until the closing of the Shanghai Sanitarium in 1949, mission work in China was a challenge. The country's leaders welcomed the missionaries' medical services, and hundreds of patients lined up daily at Adventist hospitals, dispensaries and clinics. At the same time, political turmoil, primitive living conditions, poor transportation, crime, disease, poverty and suspicion of foreigners hindered the church's mission to China.

While many Adventist physicians served this part of the world during the first half of the 20th century, the name of Harry Miller, known by many as the "China Doctor," stands above the rest. In over 70 years of service, he helped establish some 35 sanitariums and hospitals in China, the Philippines, Taiwan and Hong Kong. A humble missionary physician, Miller served high government officials and their families, as well as orphans. His introduction of a palatable soymilk that could be preserved helped save thousands of babies, and until his death in 1977, he was involved in developing soybean-based foods.

Miller's story begins at a camp meeting in the late 1890s. There he met Dr. Daniel Kress, who encouraged him to attend American Medical Missionary College at Battle Creek. He enrolled in the school's fourth class and graduated in 1902.

After graduation, he and his physician bride, Maude, felt called to serve in China— notwithstanding Dr. John Harvey Kellogg's efforts to discourage them. Along with Drs. Arthur and Bertha Selmon, and two nurses, Carrie Erickson and Charlotte Simpson, the Millers sailed across the Pacific in 1903 to join the handful of missionaries already in China.

The young doctors and nurses spent one year learning the Chinese language and way of life. After attempting formal language instruction, they found the best school was the local market. They also adopted Chinese clothing and hairstyles, and sometimes painted their faces with iodine. The men even shaved their heads except for a small patch in the back to which they each added a "pigtail" until their own hair grew long enough to braid. Miller did not cut his until he went home in 1907.

After about a year the Selmons and Millers split up and established two mission stations. Because Miller had brought a printing press from the United States, he and Maude moved near a railroad. In addition to treating patients, they printed and distributed Christian literature, thus beginning another of Miller's contributions to Christian missions. In addition to heading the Adventist publishing work in China for several years, he also served for a time as president of the church's China Division.

Tragically, Maude died of sprue in 1905. Despite pleas from family and friends to return to the United States, Miller remained in China, choosing to serve where he believed he could best fulfill God's purpose for his life.

Working in very primitive conditions, Miller often performed surgeries outdoors. He and his co-workers knew what it was to be robbed, travel hundreds of miles by mule cart, live in beggars' dens and suffer from body lice, typhus and malaria. If that weren't enough, political unrest continually interrupted their work.

When Miller returned to the United States on his first furlough, well-meaning family and friends had lined up several potential companions for him. However, he insisted that the future Mrs. Miller must also "marry" China. This turned out to be Marie Iverson, who accompanied him to Shanghai in 1907.

The Millers rented a place owned by an American-educated man with three sons and three daughters. They befriended this family, and Miller was their physician for many years. The daughters later become three of China's most famous women: Madame H.H. Kung, Madame Sun Yat-sen, and Madame Chiang Kai-shek. These and other friendships helped open doors for Adventist healthcare in China. In fact, Chang Hsueh-liang, known as the "Young Marshall" of Manchuria, provided funds for three sanitariums, two of them in appreciation for Miller's helping him overcome an opium addiction. General Chiang Kai-shek also assisted in funding the Wuhan Sanitarium in Hankow.

Only three years after returning to Shanghai, Miller became ill and had to leave China in 1911—not realizing that he would spend the next 14 years in the United States. As soon as he recovered, he assumed responsibility for the church's worldwide medical work and also became superintendent of the Washington Sanitarium in Takoma Park, Maryland. During this time he took advanced studies in thyroid surgery, a procedure that would earn him international recognition.

When Miller returned to China in 1925 to build a sanitarium in Shanghai, he found many things had changed. Sun Yat-sen had recently died, leaving the government in the hands of Chiang Kai-shek, who sought to unify the country under his nationalist organization. Instead, China would be mired in political controversy until it finally fell to communism in 1949.

Under Miller's leadership, Adventist medical work grew in China. At one time, there were nearly 20 Adventist hospitals in the country. The queen of them all was the 250-bed Shanghai Sanitarium. Miller invited Elisabeth Redelstein, a co-worker from the Washington Sanitarium, to develop a school of nursing. The Shanghai school attracted students from all over the Far East.

China Nurse

Like Miller, Redelstein made many friends in China, among them the Madame Chiang Kai-shek. While visiting her mother, a frequent sanitarium guest, she often stopped by Redelstein's office and the friendship developed.

In a rather unusual turn of events, Redelstein left the sanitarium for nine months to work for the Madame, who had accompanied her husband to a village near the Tibet border. When members of her family and staff became ill, she wrote to Miller requesting Redelstein's services. The Shanghai nurse soon found the problem: a kitchen overrun with flies and cobwebs, food left uncovered or stored in a filthy icebox, and about 20 bodyguards bathing, shaving and brushing their teeth at the sink.

Although she soon wiped out the health problem, Redelstein did not return to Shanghai right away. First she accompanied the Madame's family to a mountain retreat. Then she went with them to Nanking, where, with her knowledge of German, French and English, she often assisted the General when he entertained foreign diplomats and officers.

Just when Redelstein thought she could go back to Shanghai, the Madame requested that Miller allow her to accompany her sister, Madame Chang Hsueh-liang, to England. The wife of China's Young Marshall wished to visit her children who were studying in England, and she needed an English-speaking companion to manage travel arrangements, accommodations and meals, as well as a staff of drivers, cooks and household helpers. As it turned out, this assignment stretched to nearly nine months when one of the boys nearly died following an appendectomy.

Long-distance Prayer Circle

Madame Chang Hsueh-liang was beside herself with worry over her son. She had traveled to Paris with her children when the boy required an emergency appendectomy. Now he lay near death from resulting complications. The mother begged Redelstein to contact Dr. Miller at the Shanghai Sanitarium. She was sure he had some method that the doctors in Paris did not know.

Redelstein explained that the doctor was sailing to China and could not be reached—but yes, he had another method, a Christian method. She told her how Dr. Miller and his staff would kneel and pray to God in heaven.

"I know many, many people have been healed that way," she said.

The Buddhist woman agreed that it would be good for the Christians to pray for her son. Redelstein cabled Shanghai explaining the situation and requesting the sanitarium staff's prayers. That night the crisis passed, and the young man soon recovered.

From England, Redelstein visited her family in Germany, not realizing that the world political situation would prevent her from returning to China. With the Japanese invasion in 1937, all missionaries left the country and the Adventist medical facilities closed. Redelstein worked in Germany as a translator for the Nuremberg trials. When that work was finished, she returned to the Washington Sanitarium and Hospital, never dreaming she would ever work with the famous China Doctor again.

Meanwhile, Miller returned to the United States where he devoted his attention to developing soy-bean-based foods. Thinking to rebuild the Shanghai Sanitarium after World War II, at the age of 70, he returned to China in 1949. However, the country fell to the communists a few months after his arrival and he had to leave—this time for good.

Assuming his mission to Asia was finished, Miller again turned his attention to nutritional research, but not for long. In 1953 his good friend and fellow China missionary Ezra Longway suggested building a hospital in Taiwan, the island where China's nationalist leaders fled in 1949. Miller accepted the invitation, and soon he and Longway had raised the funds for the Taiwan Adventist Hospital. Madame Chiang Kai-shek was among the participants at the grand opening in 1955.

Once again Miller needed someone to start a school of nurses. Who else would he turn to but his friend Redelstein at the Washington Sanitarium? When she said that perhaps Taiwan was not the place for a 63-year-old nurse, Miller reminded her that he was more than 10 years her senior and age had not stopped him. Redelstein went to Taiwan, remaining there until she retired in 1959.

Miller returned to the United States in 1956—occasionally taking time from his research projects to serve as an overseas relief physician. Meanwhile, Chinese refugees were fleeing into Hong Kong by the thousands, straining the island's healthcare facilities. To help relieve the situation, Miller, now over 80, and his friend Longway, over 70, again responded to the needs of their beloved Chinese people. They located a site near the China border and raised funds for the 100-bed Tsuen Wan Hospital, which opened in 1965.

Sometime after Tsuen Wan Hospital opened, Chan Shun, owner of a large shirt manufacturing company in Hong Kong, promised Miller $1 million toward building a hospital for the island's wealthy population. The local mission agreed to the project and chose to build it on Stubbs Road, near Hong Kong's famous Victoria Peak. In 1972, at age 93, Dr. Miller was among those at the opening of his last hospital project, the 104-bed Hong Kong Adventist Hospital.

Publicity Blitz

A week or so after the Stubbs Road hospital in Hong Kong was finished, I got a call in the Far Eastern Division office. They desperately needed help up there. They had a new hospital but no patients. Nothing had been done to let the community know the hospital was open. So I went up there for a couple of months.

The first thing we did was to get a brochure together. I got it out in two days—took pictures, got them developed, wrote the copy. It was a hurriedly put together thing. Then while the printer was working on it, I got on the phone and started calling community organizations—Rotary clubs, garden clubs, any organization that would take Harry Miller as a speaker.

He'd never done this before, but he was so well known in Hong Kong, it was easy getting appointments. I'd meet him downtown at his clinic, and when he finished seeing patients, we'd go to these meetings. He'd speak, and I'd hand out the brochures. We also had an open house for news people, which produced a lot of good coverage in both English and Chinese papers.

During my two months working with Dr. Miller, we visited many offices and organizations. I remember fighting crowded city streets, trudging up and down stairways, riding elevators, and talking with people as we worked our way down a long list of people and places to visit. At the end of the day, I'd be exhausted, but not Dr. Miller. I'd watch in amazement as he briskly walked to the Star Ferry, waved me a cheery farewell, and started his hour-long trek by ferry, bus, and on foot to his home at Clearwater Bay in the New Territories.

The next morning he'd be at his office in the Man Yee Building. Sometimes he'd bring a little plastic bag containing a sample of his latest food experiment. After we'd work all day, he'd go into his laboratory at night and experiment with soy-based foods. Then he'd want me to try it. I was honest with him. If it was good, I'd tell him. When I thought it was lousy, I'd tell him. Then he'd go back and change the ingredients.

My most unforgettable moment with Dr. Miller took place just before I headed home to Singapore. He had left a clinic full of patients to meet me at the Star Ferry. (He had another sample for me to try.) In that crowded thoroughfare, we bowed our heads for a short prayer. I placed my arm around his stooped shoulders and prayed, "Thank you, God, for allowing me to know Dr. Harry Miller." —DON ROTH, ASSISTANT SECRETARY AND COMMUNICATION DIRECTOR, FAR EASTERN DIVISION OF SEVENTH-DAY ADVENTISTS, 1965–1975

SOURCES

Moore, Raymond S., *China Doctor,* Mountain. View, California: Pacific Press Publishing Association, 1969.

Ogle, Mary S., *China Nurse*, Mountain View, California: Pacific Press Publishing Association, 1974.

Roth, D.A., "The 'China Doctor'—Medical Missionary Extraordinary," *Review and Herald*, December 26, 1974.

Interviews: Marie Baldwin, Marvyn Baldwin, Gertrude Green and Don Roth.

Chapter 25

ASIA—A Thousand Miracles Every Day

No Light Matter

The Yencheng Sanitarium never had running water, and in 1939 we had electricity only three hours a week. The rest of the time we operated the whole hospital without electricity. If it was a dark day, we moved the operating table close to a window. Nurses carried kerosene lamps or candles to care for patients at night. —GERTRUDE GREEN

When Dr. Harry Miller needed a missionary nurse in China, he went to one of his Battle Creek classmates, Dr. Wells Allen Ruble at the New England Sanitarium in Massachusetts. Reluctantly, Ruble suggested his office nurse, Gertrude Green. He knew she was well qualified for overseas service with advanced training in obstetrical nursing, plus training and experience in X-ray, anesthesia and the emergency room.

However, it took a personal visit by a church official to the young nurse's mother before she accepted Miller's invitation. With her mother's blessing, she packed her textbooks, clothes and anything else she imagined she would need in China, and arrived at the Shanghai Sanitarium shortly before Christmas 1936. Before long, she would face the grim realities of mission life in China as nationalists and communists battled for control of the government, and Japan sought to make the country part of the Japanese Empire.

Green was in language study in Kuling when Japan began bombing the area in 1937. Although most of the missionaries had gone to Hong Kong or Manila, she had stayed behind with Marvin and Gertrude Loewen, who were expecting their second child. Within a few days Mrs. Loewen delivered a nine-pound boy, but tragically, the baby died within hours of birth.

A few days later Green and the Loewens walked to their mission station. To their surprise, Miller stopped to see them on his way to the Wuhan Sanitarium in Hankow. Needless to say, he was surprised to see Green.

"Pack your things," he said. "You're going with me."

The Wuhan Sanitarium was still under construction but people were already coming, including many wounded soldiers. Miller needed a good nurse to help care for them. Although Green arrived safely in Hankow, her trunk did not. Everything she had brought to help in her missionary work—textbooks, notes, clothes and bedding—was gone. It was a great loss for the young missionary, but in years to come, she would learn to get along without many things professional nurses and teachers consider essential.

Although the sanitarium had no patient beds, within a few days Green was caring for hundreds of wounded soldiers. She assisted physicians, gave anesthesia and cared for patients during the day, and stayed up late at night making surgery linens on a hand-crank sewing machine. When Japan finally took the city, she went to Hong Kong until it was safe to return.

Long Journey to Yencheng

Among Green's most memorable experiences was her 1939 move from Shanghai to central China, where she would be in charge of the school of nursing and nursing service at the Yencheng Sanitarium. Traveling with her were Dr. Winston Nethery, medical director, a Chinese lab technician, and Thelma Smith (mission treasurer) and her young son. The trip took two weeks by train and bicycle.

Before leaving Shanghai, they bought huge quantities of food and supplies, which with their personal belongings and bicycles, amounted to 190 pieces of baggage weighing more than 10,000 pounds. They shipped huge orders of flour, canned fruits and vegetables, and medical supplies by train, and would claim them at the end of the railroad, about mid-way between Shanghai and Yencheng. Then they would hire coolies to haul everything the last 250 miles.

Finding suitable accommodations along the way was a challenge. Green remembered one rat-infested place with rope beds, straw mats and thread-bare blankets that had been put on for the season and clearly used many times. The next night they stayed in a geisha house. Even though they lay awake much of the night listening to the Japanese girls serenading their customers, it was far better than the previous accommodations. Each night brought a new challenge to find lodging.

"We stayed with the chickens—any old place. Many of the Chinese had never seen white people. We were a spectacle!" Green recalled.

Finally they reached Yencheng, and while it lacked such modern conveniences as electricity and running water, the mission was on a beautiful location along the Has River. The facility consisted of three

*separate buildings, one each for male and female patients and another
for outpatients.*

~

Because World War II prevented her from returning to China after
her furlough in 1941, Green completed a baccalaureate degree and
worked in the United States until 1946. Then she returned to Yencheng,
only to find the place in shambles. Windows and doors were blown out of
any buildings left standing, and some buildings were completely
destroyed. Wasting no time, she and another staff member traveled by
freight car to pick up free building materials available from a United
Nations organization. They returned four days later with everything from
window glass to an X-ray machine.

Green had a full schedule at Yencheng, beginning with an early
morning worship service for the students, most of whom were male in
those days, followed by classes and anything but routine nursing
supervision.

"I filled in doing whatever had to be done," she said. This meant
giving anesthesia, taking X-rays, setting broken bones and even removing
bladder stones.

Green said all of her service in China was interrupted by war. In her
first term, it was the Japanese invasion, and next it would be the civil war
between Chiang Kai-shek's nationalists and Mao Tse-tung's communists.
By December 1947, the fighting was so close to Yencheng that she feared
for the safety of the hospital and mission personnel. Two church officials,
M.C. Warren and O.G. Erich, came to plan for a possible evacuation.
However, even before they had time to meet, the campus was awakened
by gunshots in the middle of the night.

Immediately, Green, Warren, Erich and three other missionaries still
remaining at Yencheng, along with about 50 Chinese women and
children, prepared to leave for Hankow where they could stay at the
Wuhan Sanitarium. The trip usually took only a few hours by train.

Angels Working Overtime

*While Green changed her clothes, something impressed her to put on
a long fur-lined Chinese dress, pants and boots. Then she packed as many
necessities as she could carry, and by 4 p.m. she and the others were at the
train station. Seven hours later the train arrived already full with people
standing in the aisles. Everything was in a state of confusion. Even
officials from the Bank of China were there will crates of money.*

Finally Green and her companions squeezed on board. Several hours passed before the train moved, and then it went only to the next village—where it remained for two days. Having thought they would be in Hankow within a matter of hours, they were hungry, cold and tired from standing.

Some time earlier, Green had befriended some Jehovah's Witnesses missionaries from this village, and suggested that Warren should try to find them. Fortunately, he did, and they graciously invited the Adventists to their mission.

Green later learned that the detained train had been a blessing in disguise for a bomb had been placed under each car. Had the train moved, they all would have died.

❧

After five days, the missionaries decided to take a coal train back to Yencheng. On a cold snowy night, they climbed onto the open car, being careful not to make any noise that could be detected by soldiers hiding in the area. The night passed, but the train never moved. About dawn, the engineer started shouting for them to get off the train.

"The communists are coming right now!" he yelled.

Everybody jumped to the ground and ran as fast as they could, not stopping until they had reached the next village nearly a mile away. There they found a Lutheran mission where they were invited to stay in a vacated house.

"It was empty except for an old pump organ in the living room," Green said. "All of us stayed in one small room. We slept on the floor and were grateful for that."

Music to Their Ears

The next morning five armed communist officers entered the mission and came to the house where the missionaries were staying. From her hiding place, Green could hear them interrogating Warren. They asked about the organ and he said it made music. They wanted a demonstration. After a moment, Warren called for her.

"Gertrude, come and play the organ."

Frightened, shaking, and clutching her Chinese songbook, she sat before the instrument while the officers pointed their guns at her as if expecting some trick. She began playing the first song she came to, and Erich started singing. Pretty soon the officers relaxed and lowered the guns. They smiled, complimented Green and then left. Sighing a prayer of thanksgiving, she looked at the words on the page before her: "Under His

Wings I am safely abiding.... I know He will keep me.... Sheltered, protected, no evil can harm me...."

The group kept moving, sometimes running from one end of a village only minutes before communist soldiers entered the other. For a short time they stayed at a Lutheran hospital compound where nationalist soldiers operated a communication facility. At night, when the fighting was most intense, they hid in a fruit cellar—unaware that it was also being used to store ammunition.

Seeing that they had no food, a supply officer gave them some flour, which they mixed with water to make "congee." Green took some of the wallpaper-paste-like mixture and made crackers.

"They had no taste, but at least it was something different," she said.

Mysterious Silence

With the nationalists losing ground to the communists, the officer advised the missionaries to move to the hospital basement. Again they huddled in a small dark place, trying to sleep amid the sounds of bombs and gunfire. Then suddenly the noise stopped. Later they learned that the communists had seen a huge army coming over the hill behind the hospital—an army much larger than theirs. The frightened soldiers threw up a flare, waved a white flag and retreated. Green fully believed God sent that army, and once again protected their small group from harm.

The next morning Green and Warren found wounded soldiers lying all over the mission compound, many of them badly hurt. Although there was little the missionaries could do to help them, Green remembered her crackers.

"We gave them all we had," she said.

Finally, a trip that usually took only a few hours on an overnight train, ended six weeks later in late January 1948. Reflecting on the experience many years later, Green said she saw God's hand in a thousand miracles every day.

SOURCES

Moore, Raymond S., *China Doctor*, Mountain View, California, Pacific Press Publishing Association, 1961.

Ogle, Mary S., *In Spite of Danger*, Washington, D.C.: Review and Herald Publishing Association, 1969.

Interview: Gertrude Green.

Chapter 26

ASIA—Land of Morning Calm

Millions Flee to Safety

Korea was anything but calm in December 1950 as 10 million people fled from the North Korea invasion. People packed into freight cars heading south, some riding on top of boxcars in the frigid winter weather. The 200-mile train ride from Seoul to Pusan took about two weeks, and December 1950 was one of the coldest in history. Dr. George Rue personally helped more than 1,200 leave Seoul. He said the hardest thing he ever did during his 40 years in Korea was to select those he could help escape to safety.

By 1950 Rue had already served the people of Korea for more than 20 years, having arrived in 1929 to reopen the work begun by Dr. Riley Russell in 1908. Russell had started in a one-room, thatch-roofed building in Soonan, and by the time he left in 1922, he had developed an 18-bed hospital. Although several other doctors followed him, each remained only a short while—one for less than 24 hours. That changed with Rue. Except for a break during World War II, he served the people of Korea continuously until 1968. He returned in 1973 to raise funds to rebuild Seoul Adventist Hospital, and during this time he shared the following stories from his experience as a missionary in Korea.

Mum's the Word

When he agreed to go to Korea in 1928, Rue insisted that it must be kept secret until after he had sold his medical practice.

"Don't worry," the gentleman from church headquarters told him. "Not a word will be said."

Early the next morning Rue received a telegram from Washington, D.C.: GLAD YOU ACCEPTED CALL TO KOREA. Immediately he hurried to the local Western Union office, and pleaded with the man who had received the message not to tell anyone. Fortunately, this man kept the secret.

Rue found things in Soonan were pretty much as Russell had left them—still no electricity or running water. He wasted no time before seeing patients on his first day in the mission field. His schedule never did allow much time for language study, but that didn't matter to the Koreans. Rue cared for them and that was enough.

Passing the Test

To practice medicine in Korea, which was then part of the Japanese Empire, physicians had to pass a licensure examination administered in Japan. The month-long process required candidates to wait for the results of one exam before taking the next. While easily passing the first set of tests, Rue felt unprepared for the last exam, the eye. Even though he had studied thoroughly and memorized pictures of eye disorders, he entered the examination hall feeling ill prepared.

Here he faced 15 to 20 persons, each with a different eye disorder. The examiner directed him to the first. It was a perfect textbook example and Rue identified it correctly. Then he went to the next person. This too was a textbook example, as were the third and fourth cases. The examination continued until Rue had identified each case and passed the examination with high scores.

While most missionary work was restricted, there was always a need for medical care. In 1931 Rue moved to Seoul, and opened a clinic in an old pottery factory. Patients immediately began coming, but Rue could not admit them to local hospitals because of closed medical staffs. In spite of this, patients continued coming until he was crowded for space. To help the situation, he moved into a Japanese-style building large enough for nine patients. That facility continued operation until late 1937.

A Car Would Help

Rue was not shy about asking for donations to help his work in Korea. Transportation was one of the big inconveniences. Although another missionary had a Model A Ford, he never used it, and Rue could hardly stand knowing that car sat idle in a garage. Finally he persuaded the owner to sell it to him. Then he persuaded some friends in the United States to send him the money to pay for it.

With a successful clinic underway, plans began in 1934 to build a permanent hospital on a rural site outside Seoul. Before the building was finished, a friend from the city came to look over the facility, and gave

$1,000 for a TB room. Unfortunately, the money ran out before the room was done. The donor had no more cash to give, but he offered the doctor a two-year-old car with a V-8 engine. Rue happily took it and sold his Model A. He was among the first to drive a private car in Korea, as evidenced by his auto license number 29.

The hospital opened in January 1936. Sadly, about Christmastime that same year, Mrs. Rue died from complications following surgery. While others might have returned home after such a tragedy, Rue stayed. He often said, "My life belongs to Korea."

Short-wave Reports

Returning from a picnic one afternoon in October 1940, Rue learned that missionaries were being evacuated from Korea, Manchuria and China. He immediately thought of his children, Betty and George, Jr., who were attending school in Shanghai. As it turned out, they and other students from the Adventist academy were already on a ship headed to the United States. Before crossing the Pacific Ocean, however, it stopped at Korea, giving Rue a chance to see his children.

For nearly a month he awaited news that they had arrived in the United States. Although it was illegal in Korea for civilians to own short-wave radios, Rue had one. He listened every night to keep abreast of war developments and news from home. One Sunday night the announcer read a short message addressed to GHR: "Your children arrived safely. They were met by their aunt and uncle and are on their way to Loma Linda."

Finally in the spring of 1941, church officials advised Rue to leave Korea. The local staff continued operating the hospital until the Japanese took it over in 1943 and turned it into a tuberculosis facility.

Rue worked in the States until he could return to Korea. During this time he married Grace Lea, a registered nurse. Also, his daughter married Lee Mitchell, a teacher at the Adventist college near Seoul. George and Lee were informed in 1946 that they could return to Korea. However, the paperwork and travel arrangements took five months, so they didn't arrive in Seoul until March 1947.

Under Rue's leadership, the Seoul Sanitarium and Hospital drew patients from all walks of life. The doctor usually worked 16 hours a day, often seeing as many as 250 patients a day—notwithstanding frequent power blackouts. After one late-night power failure during surgery, he made sure a flashlight was always on the tray with his surgical instruments.

Unfortunately, the end of World War II did not mean peace for Korea. Communists in the north proclaimed a People's Republic in 1948 with the intention of making Seoul their capital. The south responded by formalizing the Republic of South Korea and making Syngman Rhee president.

During this time, the U.S. State Department reserved beds at various mission hospitals for possible use by Americans. In exchange the hospitals received help to rebuild and add equipment. While the Adventist hospital set aside 15 beds for this purpose, they were seldom used, and Rue was not pleased when the State Department wanted to increase the number.

"You've got 15 and you don't use them," he protested.

Offering no further explanation, the officials insisted on the additional beds, and provided materials to expand the hospital.

Startling News

Rue attended the Adventist church's 1950 General Conference session in San Francisco, leaving Korea ahead of his wife to attend an American Medical Association meeting. When people asked about the war in Korea, he assured them that the radio and television reports were greatly exaggerated. Obviously, no one was more surprised than he when the June 25 evening news reported the fall of Seoul. He sat in his brother-in-law's living room in Napa, California, watching television in disbelief and wondering where his wife was.

Back in Korea, Mrs. Rue had fled to Inchon and boarded a Norwegian fertilizer ship bound for Japan with about 500 other Americans. Some in the group, including Irene Robson, director of nursing at the Adventist hospital, would remain in Japan until they could return to Korea. Mrs. Rue continued on to the United States.

Not knowing how long he would be in the States, Rue sold his car to the U.S. Embassy in Seoul, and took classes at the Mayo Clinic in Minnesota. That's where he was when General Douglas MacArthur and the United Nations troops landed in Inchon on September 15, 1950, and 11 days later recaptured Seoul.

In early October President Rhee asked Rue to return to Seoul, and this time there was no waiting. The process that had taken five months in 1947 took only two hours in 1950. Arriving in Seoul, the Rues found the hospital badly damaged. Their house was nearly empty and what little remained was beyond repair.

"We looked around and found an old piece of carpet covered with weeds. We threw it over some box springs, and that's where we slept," he said.

Nurse Robson joined the Rues in Korea, but she was the last Adventist missionary allowed into the country at that time. As the war intensified, the doctor began evacuating hospital workers and church members to Pusan. He bought back his V-8 automobile, and the U.S. Embassy gave him a jeep and three-quarter-ton truck to use. He was also notified when the embassy had a freight car going to Pusan, and he could usually send about a dozen people on it.

Finally all Americans were ordered out of Seoul. Robson and Mrs. Rue flew to Pusan in an embassy plane, while Dr. Rue went later by truck. Being among the last to leave, he volunteered to help alert people around the city of the mandatory evacuation. One of his last stops was the hospital boiler room. After instructing the attendant to open the valve and drain the heating system, the doctor stopped at his house to get some blankets and then went to the embassy to catch his ride to Pusan.

The embassy vehicles departed at exactly 5:40 p.m.—13 cars and two trucks with oil, gasoline and as many other provisions as they could carry. All was on schedule until they reached the Han River, where the main bridge had been destroyed. One pontoon bridge was handling two lines of traffic headed south and three lines of military vehicles headed north. The embassy vehicles crossed the river around 10 p.m.—only a few hours before North Korea took Seoul.

Separated Again

After finding his wife and Robson in the nurses' barracks at the evacuation hospital in Pusan, Rue went to the Army officer's mess hall to get something to eat and find a place to stay. All persons eating in the mess hall had to sign in and indicate their units. Rue simply signed "SDA" after his name, and was never questioned during the two months he ate there. Finding a bed, however, was not so easy. He stayed in a number of places, moving every couple of weeks.

Pusan, a town of 250,000, was not equipped to feed and shelter two million people. While some refugees were relocated, the Adventist group stayed together, crowded inside two small churches and a tent. Rue didn't know what to do with them until he overheard some officers discussing the refugee problem and the lack of medical help on Cheju Island. He politely interrupted them.

"I've got all the help you need," he said.

Room for More

Arrangements were soon underway to take most of the Adventists to Cheju. Rue asked a couple of men to make a list of names and tell his group when and where to catch the ship. As it turned out, they never compiled the list, but when news of the ship going to Cheju spread, 5,000 people showed up and crowded on board. Rue had no idea which ones were in his group. Although under strong protest from ship officials, the doctor even took his jeep and truck.

సా

On Cheju Island, the hospital group set up a clinic. Robson organized the nurses, who gave thousands of inoculations for typhoid, cholera and smallpox.

When a story hit the news that a woman had given birth on the Han River Bridge one cold morning in January 1951, President Rhee told his wife to find Rue and set up a hospital as quickly as possible. With the city overflowing with refugees, where would they find a vacant building? Finally they located a barn-like structure with one large room measuring about 17 feet by 24 feet—big enough for 16 patients.

"It wasn't much, but it was all we could find, and we made it work," Rue said.

He converted the building into the Pusan Branch of the Seoul Sanitarium and Hospital and initially provided free care. Only the nursery had stationary walls, with patient rooms and departments separated by hanging bed sheets. Rue performed several surgeries here until the Pusan Adventist Hospital opened in 1955.

Housing the staff in Pusan in 1951 was a huge challenge. A few lived in huts behind the main structure. Four couples, some with children, stayed in a large tent divided by curtains into four tiny "apartments." They lived there nearly three years, and the doctor said he never heard a complaint.

The Seoul Sanitarium and Hospital reopened in 1951, having suffered severe damage in the war. Thousands of dollars worth of supplies and equipment were lost, and the nurses' dormitory was burned. Also, in the excitement of closing down operations during the evacuation, the man in the boiler room had failed to turn off the valve, resulting in broken pipes and extensive water damage.

However, all the hospital records were recovered, thanks to employees who had buried them in the surrounding hills. While bombs and fires destroyed much of the area, the medical and financial records had been safely preserved.

When it came to rebuilding the Seoul Sanitarium, the U.S. government provided trucks, cement mixers, gravel, sand and other construction materials in addition to funds. The Adventist church gave $20,000, and another $10,000 came from a Christmas offering to help the various church-sponsored hospitals in Seoul. Gradually, additional missionaries came to staff the hospital, school and church headquarters.

Another Mission Calls

One of the tragedies of the Korean War was the large number of orphans, many of them left at the hospital. Mrs. Rue set up an orphanage in 1951, which cared for over 1,000 children until it closed in the 1970s. Many of the children were adopted, but several remained at the orphanage and trained at the hospital's school of nursing or Korean Union College.

SOURCES

Kim, Penny, unpublished manuscript, 1998.

Rue, George H., tape recordings, 1974.

Chapter 27

ASIA—Opportunities in India

Abandoned Hunt

India's big cats would come out at night looking for an unsuspecting cow or goat or a careless wild pig rooting in a peanut patch. A farmer's cow might easily be worth the equivalent of his annual income, so locals always knew the whereabouts of Mr. Leopard and Mr. Stripes and kept their livestock at a safe distance.

Religious beliefs prohibited the villagers from killing the big cats and other predators, but Christian missionaries were permitted to own guns and they could do the deadly deed. In the early 1920s, long before missionary teacher Theodore Flaiz had studied medicine or dreamed of heading the church's worldwide healthcare work, both he and his wife saved more than one farmer's livelihood with a deadly shot.

Years later Dr. Dunbar Smith set out to test his aim on a big cat that had become a neighborhood nuisance. He devised a seemingly foolproof plan, although it put the family's pet goat Mutton Currie at ultimate risk.

Like Abraham leading Isaac to the sacrificial altar, Smith led Mutton Currie into the jungle and tied him to a tree. Then the doctor climbed up and sat on a strong limb from which he would have a clear shot when the cat came prowling for a late night meal. However, when he reached down to get the gun from his assistant, the weapon went off accidentally, sending a bullet whirring past his head. Thus ended Smith's tiger hunt—no doubt to the great relief of Mutton Currie!

India was among the first destinations for Adventist missionaries, with some arriving in the 1890s to establish work near Calcutta. Here they encountered many diseases, epidemics and other health problems, and whether they were medically trained or not, they provided whatever treatments they could. During smallpox and cholera epidemics, early missionaries devoted nearly all of their time to caring for the sick.

Soon after Dr. Herman Menkel's arrival in 1907, the main Adventist medical work in India moved north to a cooler climate in the foothills of the Himalayas. Originally, this place was used as a retreat for missionaries needing relief from the intense heat of the lowlands. The Simla

Sanitarium began here in 1915 and, except between 1943 and 1950, has remained open.

Adventists owned numerous medical facilities in India over the years, but many of them closed for various reasons, ranging from financial failure to political problems. Among those remaining in operation today is Ranchi Adventist Hospital at Bihar, established in 1949 by Dr. R.V. Shearer, who converted a school and office building into a healthcare facility. Also, Ruby Nelson Memorial Hospital in Punjab—named for a missionary who was murdered in India—opened in 1965. Today this hospital specializes in ophthalmology. The well-equipped Ottapalam Seventh-day Adventist Hospital in north Kerala, established in 1969, serves a rural but thickly populated area. For about 10 years Dr. Mary Small, whom some call the "Mother Teresa of Ottapalam," practiced obstetrics and gynecology here. Of her experience, she said her greatest challenge was professional loneliness. She missed opportunities to consult with other specialists and attend professional conferences.

Dr. Dunbar Smith, minister and physician in India, Sri Lanka and Burma (Myanmar) between 1939–1956, provided some of the following stories from Adventist healthcare in India:

During the 1920s, a local landowner—known as a zamindar—wanted a hospital for the people of his region. Dr. Flaiz, then mission superintendent, negotiated the deal in which the landowner gave the Adventists five acres of land, three uncompleted buildings and cash to build a hospital. At the zamindar's request, the new hospital was named in honor of an officer in the British India Army.

The 21-bed Giffard Memorial Hospital opened in 1925 and grew to 45 beds by 1942. When it closed for a while during World War II, a handful of local workers operated a dispensary. Then in 1944, Dr. Elizabeth Hiscox reopened the hospital and served there for 42 years. Scores of other missionaries also served at Giffard Memorial Hospital, some of them for many years.

One-stop Services

"Dr. Hiscox would tackle anything. When closing the incision, while a patient was still anesthetized, we opened his mouth and extracted all the diseased teeth and remaining roots. Sometimes, while recovering, the patient wondered why his mouth was as sore as his abdomen. There was no extra charge!"

Until the mid-1950s, Giffard's doctors and nurses worked without air-conditioning. Smith, who served there for about a year, remembers one summer when his family and the other missionaries had taken a customary vacation or "hill leave." On this particular occasion, he remained behind to care for patients.

Long Hot Days

"I was alone. The temperature during several weeks went up to 117 degrees every day," writes Smith. "After morning inspection of the hospital, patients, and clinic—during which I might see 100 patients—I went my weary way home, ate a bite of dinner, and prepared to rest. I placed a charpoy, sort of a cot, in the front room under the electric fan, poured a bucket of water over [the charpoy] *and over me and lay down. Shortly, I would awaken, profusely perspiring with the water all evaporated and the fan blasting hot air upon me. Then I would repeat the process. At four in the afternoon I would return to the hospital, see more patients, check on the inpatients, and be home by seven or eight."*

∾

Not surprisingly, the employees' homes were soon wired for electricity and electric fans were installed in the doctors' offices.

Adventist medical work began in Surat, Gujarat, in 1936, when Dr. George Nelson opened a clinic. Before long residents of this area about 150 miles north of Bombay wanted a full hospital. Funds were raised, and in early 1942 a 25-bed hospital opened just outside the city.

Smith served at Surat Hospital from 1953 to 1956, working with Dr. Joelle Rentfro, whom he described as "fearless and ready to attack any medical or surgical problem." When faced with a condition that she and Smith were unfamiliar with, she would tell him to read up on it and they'd tackle it the next day.

Because Surat Hospital had the only air-conditioned operating room in that part of India in the mid-1950s, surgery was always welcome. One day Smith found the surgery room door open. Entering, he found Rentfro caring for a little girl whose hemoglobin was so low he wondered how she could live. He saw the doctor take blood from her own vein and inject it into the child's vein, in order to save her.

The life of a medical missionary in India was full of challenges, adventure and sacrifices, and sometimes, sadly, the ultimate sacrifice. Smith tells of one such incident that took the life of a missionary child. Merle Manley, principal of Vincent Hill School where many missionaries' children attended, asked Smith to examine one of the students, Billy Storz. The diagnosis was bulbar poliomyelitis.

Very Sad Day

"There was a mission hospital on the other side of Mussoorie. The doctor there agreed to take Billy, who was now unconscious. We took him over in a hammock slung from poles on the backs of coolies. The hospital had a wooden version of an iron lung, into which we put Billy. It was operated continuously by coolies, who pumped away. Tanks of oxygen were ordered from New Delhi. I looked after him during the day, while the hospital doctor on night call took care of him at night. [My wife and sister-in-law] *and nurses from our school alternated in providing care around the clock.... The government tried to locate* [Billy's] *parents by wireless.... They arrived, only to catch a glimpse of their unconscious son through a small window, before he passed away.*

"As neither Principal Manley nor the church pastor was emotionally able to take the funeral service, it fell to me. How sad, not only for the parents and fellow students, but for all. We buried him at Vincent Hill School—another sacrifice to foreign mission service."

SOURCE

Smith, Dunbar W., M.D., *The Travels, Triumphs and Vicissitudes of Dunbar W. Smith, M.D.*, Loma Linda, California: Dunbar W. Smith, M.D. 1994.

Chapter 28

ASIA—Bygone Days of Burma

Early Work in Rangoon

Adventist medical work in Myanmar, formerly Burma, began in the early 1900s. Dr. Ollie Oberholtzer started the first permanent work in 1907, and 14 years later F.A. Wyman and his wife opened treatment rooms in Rangoon. While all mission work ceased during World War II, an old Rangoon hotel was later converted into a 60-bed hospital. By 1955 it had grown to 115 beds with six physicians and 40,000 patients a year.

It was considered the best hospital in Burma and patients came from all over the country. With government changes, however, the hospital was nationalized in 1965 and all overseas missionaries left.

Eric Hare was best known as a storyteller, who for many years held children spellbound with tales from his mission experiences. For 16 years he specialized in youth programs while he was an associate in the Sabbath School Department of the General Conference of Seventh-day Adventists.

Interestingly, Hare began his career in 1915 as a missionary nurse. After studying nursing at Sydney Sanitarium in Australia, he went to Burma, where he acquired the nickname "Dr. Rabbit." At first he thought it was simply a word play on his name, but he would later learn that it had something to do with an old folk tale.

Hare was asleep in his bamboo house one night when a group of men from a nearby village awakened him. They said a woman and boy had been severely beaten and would certainly die without his help. Through the dark tiger-inhabited jungle, Hare hiked with them to their village.

He entered the house to find the woman and boy on the floor. He nearly fainted from the sight and smell of blood. Fearing the woman had already died, he began working on the boy, who had a deep gash in his neck and two fingers missing. After a while Dr. Rabbit realized that the woman was still alive. Some of the villagers left to find someone to help him, but the man they brought back fainted as soon as he came into the house. Finally an old woman offered to help. She said she was so old and skinny that the evil spirits had no interest in her and it would do no harm for her to help him.

Immediately the two went to work. The injured woman's forehead was split open. One cheek was nearly severed from her face, and her left arm had been cut off just below the elbow. Dr. Rabbit and his assistant bandaged her wounds as best they could while the village men made a bamboo stretcher to transport her 60 miles to a government hospital. He knew it would be a miracle if she lived.

Six weeks later, while Hare was caring for patients, a woman with a badly scarred face came up to him. He didn't recognize her until she pulled away her shawl and revealed the stump where her arm had been cut off. Knowing the woman's story, the other patients began reciting lines from one of their folk tales.

"Dr. Rabbit"

"Didn't the rabbit save the elephant's life when the tiger was going to eat him all up?

"Didn't the rabbit tell the horse how to get two sets of teeth so he could whinny?

"And wasn't the rabbit the best doctor?"

"Isn't this white doctor our Dr. Rabbit?

"Sure, he is our Dr. Rabbit."

ॐ

Suddenly Hare realized the significance of his nickname. With a certainty, the people he would serve for nearly 20 years had accepted him. He and his family remained in Burma until World War II, and were among those who trekked the long Burma Road to evacuate the country. During his lifetime he wrote 11 books, some 200 articles, and shared countless stories, many of them from his experience as a missionary nurse.

SOURCES

Barger, R. Curtis, *Don't You Know? Haven't You Heard? The Life Story of Eric B. Hare*, Hagerstown, Maryland: Review and Herald Publishing Association, 1985.

Interview and Notes: William Murrill.

Chapter 29

ASIA—Setting Sail for Siam

Fabulously Wealthy City

It was an unusual proposal, but Ellen Dick, a student nurse in Loma Linda, California, said yes when Dr. Ralph Waddell invited her to go with him to Bangkok. Ever since hearing of countries visited by Dr. Horace Hall, a missionary to the Philippines, Waddell had dreamed of serving in Siam's "fabulously wealthy city." Finally the young doctor's dream became reality in 1937. With their four-month-old daughter, the Waddells set sail for Siam to establish Adventist healthcare in Thailand.

Waddell and leaders of the Siam Mission wasted no time. They found a suitable site for a clinic in a row of shop houses where residents lived on the second floor and operated small businesses or industries on the ground level. After moving 40 families and renovating the building, Waddell opened the 12-bed Mission Clinic. Within days all beds were occupied and the doctor soon had to find ways to expand, sometimes in most unconventional ways.

Most of the Siamese feared the spirits of the dead. Whenever they heard that a patient had died, residents of the adjacent shop houses would move out and the clinic would move in. To encourage expansion, Waddell even set up the morgue along a wall adjacent to the next shop house.

Solution for Unusual Problem

At one time, several ladies of the night set up shop next to the clinic. This posed no problem until some of them were discovered on the second floor ledge, soliciting patients. Waddell knew exactly what to do.

"We placed a small dish of dilute hydrochloric acid with a bit of ferrous sulphate in the common drain going to their quarters. The stench was rather unpleasant—something like rotten eggs. After three days the manager came and asked if we would like to take over her shop since she was thinking of moving elsewhere."

This made room for four more beds and a hydrotherapy department. In a short time the clinic grew to 50 beds—plus five canvas cots that could be used when needed.

Some wealthy patients encouraged the doctor to expand into a nearby "Annex," which had been the home of an English lawyer. Optimistically, Waddell leased the building and put in 30 beds. By the end of the first week every bed was full, creating a heavy workload for the small staff. However, with a total of 85 beds, the clinic qualified to operate a school of nursing, which would help alleviate the staffing crisis.

Others soon joined the Bangkok clinic, including Dr. George Innocent, Dr. Donald LaTourette and nurse Ruth Munroe, director of the school of nursing. Word of the clinic also spread to other areas. In southern Thailand, residents of Phuket invited Adventists to start a clinic on their island. Dr. Arthur Geschke responded to this opportunity in 1940.

Soon the Bangkok staff began dreaming of a large new hospital to better serve the Thai people. They planned to begin after the Waddells returned from furlough in 1941. Unfortunately, World War II brought a halt to all missionary work in Thailand.

Sounds of War

"We were awakened the morning of December 8...by planes flying overhead, an unusual sound in 1941. My husband quickly turned on the short-wave radio, and above the static [we heard] *BBC announce the startling news: Pearl Harbor had been bombed; Manila and Singapore were under attack; Japanese troops were approaching the coast of Malaysia. Within hours they would be in Bangkok!"* —ELSA LATOURETTE

The Thai staff took over responsibility for the clinic under the leadership of a young man named Nai Pleng Vitiamyalaksana, who was left with no physicians and no money to operate it. The Japanese claimed that because the Annex was an American facility, he had no right to it. Pleng finally convinced them it was an international building, and they agreed to rent it from him.

Unable to pay the staff immediately, he promised them if they worked hard and depended on the Lord, they could keep the clinic open. He hired a Romanian physician, an acquaintance of Waddell's in private practice in Bangkok, and the clinic reopened only three days after the Japanese invasion.

Mission Clinic Saved

A Japanese officer entered the clinic one day, demanding to know who owned the hospital and who managed it. Pleng told him the Thailand Mission owned it and that he, a Thai, managed it. Seeing no evidence of Americans, the officer told him to go ahead with his business. But that was not enough for Pleng.

"Just a minute," he said as the man turned to leave. "Will you please write me a note authorizing us to continue operating our hospital?"

The officer said no, but he knew who could. He took Pleng to the Ministry of Commerce, where a large group of officials were discussing the fate of private hospitals in Thailand. They had just voted to confiscate all of them, but when the Japanese officer said he had authorized Pleng to continue operations, the Mission Clinic was saved.

The clinic thrived, partly because it offered hydrotherapy, which drew dozens of patients. One was a Mr. Aoka, former mayor of Osaka, Japan, who generously paid the clinic more than enough to cover the monthly rent.

When the Waddells learned they could return to Bangkok in 1945, they began buying equipment and supplies and in no time were well over the 350-pound limit per ship passenger. They continued to shop and pack and arrived in San Francisco with over 16 tons of baggage—only to be met by a passenger agent in no mood for negotiating. Waddell had no intention of leaving even one pound of baggage behind. He pleaded with the agent, describing the dire needs of Thailand, until the man called his supervisor. After an hour or so Waddell had permission to take all 16 tons aboard.

In Bangkok, clinic workers and church members welcomed the Waddells with stories of the war and how God had preserved the medical work. They were most pleased to announce that they had saved approximately $10,000 to expand the clinic. Soon the medical effort in Bangkok was growing as rapidly as it had before the war, and plans were made to build a 100-bed hospital.

Many people played important roles in developing Adventist healthcare in Thailand, both Thais and overseas missionaries. Among them was nurse Gertrude Green, who had previously worked 10 years in China. She would serve at the Bangkok Adventist Hospital for more than 40 years.

"When I got home from China, the General Conference asked me where I wanted to go," Green recalled. "I'd had Thai students in China, and they were such nice people. I chose Bangkok."

She arrived five days before the grand opening in 1951 and immediately went to work sprucing up the hospital for the big event. With a bucket in hand, she climbed a ladder and washed the louvered windows above the doors of each patient room—much to the amazement of the Thai nurses and students. Getting ready for thousands of guests and dignitaries expected at the grand opening meant the hospital must be spotless, and she willingly did her part to make sure it made a good impression.

What a grand opening it was! Four thousand invitations were mailed. Newspapers carried announcements and stories. Indeed, the new hospital was the biggest story in the city, with such honored guests as the prime minister of Thailand, the mayor of Bangkok, ambassadors, diplomats, cabinet ministers and many others. Guests from all walks of life crowded into four large tents supplied by the Thai army. After touring the new facility, Prime Minister Pibulsonggram declared, "This is the best in Thailand!"

Golden Moment

"Our Indian watchman dressed in his new white suit and draped with a red shoulder strap bearing the word 'SANITARIUM' was at the gate directing the unending stream of traffic.

"It was my privilege to give a few words of welcome to the hundreds of guests who had come to share in the joy of opening another link in the great chain of Adventist medical institutions…. At the conclusion of my remarks, I presented the Premier to the audience and he arose to greet them amid thunderous applause. He gave a very fine address…. At this point he pulled a long, red silk ribbon which unfurled a thin veil thus displaying to the public the golden words BANGKOK SANITARIUM AND HOSPITAL." —DR. RALPH WADDELL

With the new hospital open and running, it was time for the Waddells to take another furlough. While they were gone, a coup threw the country into a state of war.

Surprise Attack

Life on the hospital campus had been perfectly normal that Friday as people prepared for the coming Sabbath. Green went to her hairdresser, but could not get a taxi or bus to take her back to the hospital.

"I came out and found the street empty," she recalled. "There were no cars, no buses. I started walking and praying. Then I saw a big military truck carrying soldiers with guns."

By the time she reached the hospital, the hallways were crowded with wounded soldiers and civilians. The staff worked day and night throughout the three-day ordeal.

ॐ

The Bangkok San grew into a strong and highly regarded organization and the school of nursing attracted many young Thais. However, because the country had a severe shortage of physicians, the government required all registered schools of nursing to offer a midwifery program. Green accepted the challenge.

From the beginning, midwifery services were to be provided as charity care, and would include health classes for the mothers. The program would provide training for the students, quality maternity care for the poor and education. A dedicated midwifery building with 24 beds was completed in December 1954. The teaching curriculum was ready, and nine students had been carefully selected. Opening ceremonies were scheduled for January 4, 1955, with the prime minister's wife to cut the ribbon. The morning of the event, Green received an unexpected phone call from the prime minister—requesting permission to attend the opening with his wife. Of course, Green was honored that he should be interested in the new department.

In time the midwifery program grew, with added nurses and faculty. Some months the staff helped deliver as many as 160 babies. Although Green personally delivered thousands of babies, when asked exactly how many, she preferred to say, "Too many."

Approximately 1,200 students went through the midwifery program during the years that Green was associated with Bangkok Adventist Hospital. The school earned an excellent reputation and became a government model for training midwifery nurses. It's not surprising that when she decided to retire at the age of 74, the hospital asked her to continue a little while longer. She did—for 12 more years!

SOURCES

Nai Pleng Vitiamyalaksana, editor, *Spray of Golden Shower: A Memory Book Commemorating the Fiftieth Anniversary of Bangkok Adventist Hospital, 1937 to 1987*, Bangkok: Thailand Publishing House of Seventh-day Adventists, 1987.

Interview: Gertrude Green.

Chapter 30

ASIA—War's End Closes Vietnam Hospital

April 1975

"All seemed to be going well until we reached the gate near the civilian terminal and a policeman boarded the bus. My heart sank when I saw him motion to the young teen-age son of our mission president, and ask for his ID card and papers. The policeman looked at me and smiled, but I did not smile back. He sent the lad back to his seat, and got off the bus. Then a helmeted ARVN soldier got on the bus and rode with us to the plane. As the bus approached the aircraft that would take us safely to Guam, I got up and stood directly back of the soldier. He turned his head slightly and spoke to me in perfect English.

"U.S. money for the policeman and me or the boy does not get on the plane."

"I dug my hand into my pocket and brought out a U.S. $10 bill. I gave it to him and he waved the young man on. When the last of our group was off the bus, the soldier gave me a brief salute, and that was the last I saw of him." —DON ROTH, RETIRED ASSOCIATE SECRETARY, GENERAL CONFERENCE OF SEVENTH-DAY ADVENTISTS

Saigon Adventist Hospital always operated in an environment of war. Civil war broke out only days before it opened in May 1955, and it served civilians throughout the Vietnam War. With the fall of the country in 1975, plans for a replacement facility never materialized. Nonetheless, for 20 years Saigon Adventist Hospital played an important role in the church's healthcare mission.

To meet the need for nurses, the hospital operated one of only two nursing schools in the country for a few years. Then nurses were recruited from Thailand and the Philippines, but as the Vietnam War intensified, it became very difficult to attract nurses from other countries. The hospital desperately needed to find a director to reactivate the school—no easy task in the 1960s. A two-year search ended in 1968 when a young woman from Texas—a graduate from the Loma Linda University School of Nursing—accepted the challenge. Marilyn Bennett (now Justesen) had been out of college less than a year and had no teaching experience when she agreed to go to Vietnam.

In Saigon she found 50 to 60 patients crammed into a 38-bed facility—a dirty old yellow building that had been a French mansion in a former life. Military convoys roared past the three-story hospital. Helicopters clattered over the mission that had witnessed the Tet Offensive a few months before her arrival. Motorcycles, taxis, trucks and "cyclos"—motorcycles equipped with a second seat on the front—buzzed, whizzed and swarmed through the dirty streets. Rock and roll music poured from nearby bars day and night. Inside the crowded hospital, people yelled in order to be heard.

Patient Overflow

"In spite of the continual commotion, the sick thronged into the hospital compound, teeming through the iron gates, pushing and shoving their way into the crowded courtyard and on into the small, packed waiting room. Here the people huddled together on long wooden benches or lay on canvas stretchers until the doctors could see them. The waiting room served as an overflow ward when the other areas of the hospital filled up. Then the outpatients sat on the floor or stood pressed in together while hospital patients filled the wooden benches. At times, bottles of intravenous fluids hung precariously from the louvered glass windowpanes, since the hospital never had enough rickety IV poles to go around. Under the wooden benches sat bedpans, a taunting reminder of the total lack of privacy. Some days the waiting room and hospital grounds were so jammed that one had to push and shove his way through." —MARILYN BENNETT

A winding staircase provided the only access between floors. Patients, equipment and supplies had to be carried up and down the stairs—a tricky maneuver on the narrow curved stairways. Some patients walked, but sometimes the physician simply carried patients to and from surgery. People were everywhere—in the hallways, on the outpatient clinic floor, on desktops and occasionally crowded two to a bed. The director of nurses once found a baby had been left in a box on her desk and another on a chair.

Patients in Saigon suffered everything from cancer to gallbladder attacks, arthritis and tuberculosis. Motorcycle accidents were so common that the staff came up with the diagnosis abbreviation HBH for "hit by Honda." When medical supplies ran short, the U.S. Army generously supplied obsolete, surplus and duplicate materials. Physicians from the nearby 3rd Field Army Hospital assisted as their time permitted.

Having no teaching experience, Bennett was overwhelmed with the responsibility of running a three-year nursing program. It involved everything from developing curriculum and teaching to recruiting faculty, laying floor tile and painting the barracks that would house student nurses and classrooms. Fortunately some good-hearted GIs assisted with labor and supplies. However, it wasn't until after the last brush stroke of Army green paint had been spread on the barracks that Bennett learned the houses of ill repute in Vietnam were painted green. She later had the building repainted an acceptable Air Force gray.

When it came to faculty, she recruited overseas missionaries, Vietnamese employees, GIs, Americans with the USAID organization, and American women whose husbands worked under military contracts.

To give her students clinical experience, she worked out affiliation privileges with seven government hospitals and the 3rd Field Hospital.

"How all by myself I ever amassed the courage to approach the commander of the 3rd Field Hospital, the chief Army nurse for the entire military in Vietnam, and finally the Surgeon General's office to get affiliation privileges remains a miraculous mystery to me," she said later.

This affiliation allowed her students to observe excellent patient care and equipment not available in other Vietnamese hospitals. Soon the school was considered the best in the country, and received 150 applications for the 15 spaces in the second class.

Blonde Bombshell

Saigon Adventist Hospital staff traveled to orphanages, schools and refugee camps to immunize children against diphtheria, whooping cough, tetanus, typhoid, cholera, plague and polio. But when requests became too numerous, a student volunteer from the United States came to direct the program. Ruthita Jensen (now Fike), nicknamed by her college classmates the "Blonde Bomb to Vietnam," arrived in 1970, and for a year she traveled in and around Saigon by helicopter, truck, car and jeep, armed with a compressed air immunization gun. She and the hospital staff vaccinated more than 100,000 children during the war.

Soon after Bennett and Jensen left Vietnam, plans were made for a 175-bed replacement facility. When the Americans began pulling out of Vietnam prior to the January 1973 cease-fire, the U.S. government offered the 3rd Field Army Hospital to the Adventists. The agreement included more than a million dollars' worth of donated equipment for the new hospital. However, the events of April 1975 ended that plan.

Just days before the South Vietnam government surrendered to communist forces, church leaders from Singapore and Saigon met to determine the fate of their work and personnel in South Vietnam. The Vietnamese were so concerned about their families they could not concentrate on saving the hospital and other church organizations. Finally the leaders decided to evacuate about 40 women and children with more to follow.

Don Roth, then assistant secretary and communication director for the Far Eastern Division of Seventh-day Adventists, volunteered to take the first group. Because three of the women were pregnant, he insisted that at least two nurses go with him.

Roth went to the American news agencies in downtown Saigon and learned from reporters that all the paperwork was being handled at the airport.

"I went out there and just walked in. It was a big old barracks kind of thing or gymnasium. They had desks all over and these guys were making out the forms. I went to the guy the reporters told me to see. He knew all about the 3rd Field Hospital. He knew that these Vietnamese would be eligible to be evacuated," says Roth.

The complicated process involved making lists of names and sponsors to be approved by the U.S. Embassy. As a sponsor, Roth had to sign an affidavit that expenses in connection with resettling each Vietnamese would be covered. Then the names had to be placed on a manifest for the aircraft.

"I was able to type up my own manifest for the flight and later helped type the manifests of other groups," says Roth, who types as fast with two fingers as most people do with 10.

When all the paper work was done and he had a flight time, he went back to the hospital to notify his group to be ready to leave Tan Son Nhut Airport in two hours. They arrived to find the place crowded with thousands of people.

Roth's group moved to the nearby recreation center for the U.S. Defense Attaché Office, where they joined about a thousand other refugees in a bowling alley. He lay down across the lanes, putting his head against his camera bag in one gutter and hanging his legs over the opposite gutter.

Destination Guam

The first flight of the day took group number 88. Roth's group, 107, was not called until 3 p.m. While his people boarded a C-141 cargo jet, he helped load the baggage. When the huge back door slammed shut, Roth found a place to sit, leaned back and looked at the scene around him.

About 70 very tired Vietnamese strapped into web seats lined each side of the aircraft, while 100 or more others sat on the floor without seat belts. There were only two small containers of water and one restroom on the aircraft.

"What a flight this is going to be," Roth thought as the plane taxied down the runway and headed for Guam. (Lucky for him, no babies were born in flight.)

࿓

A total of 450 Vietnamese from the Adventist hospital and other organizations evacuated the country over the next few days. Later the new government seized the church's hospital, publishing house and schools.

SOURCES

Bennett, Marilyn Faye, *Help! What Do I Do Now?* Nashville, Tennessee: Southern Publishing Association, 1976.

Hancock, John H., "The Fastest Gun in the—East!" *Signs of the Times*, July 1970.

Jensen, Ruthita, "Student Missionary Jensen Operates Vaccination Clinic," *Clock Tower*, Lincoln, Nebraska, 1970 or 1971.

Roth, D.A., "Adventists Take Over Army Hospital," *Australasian Record*, April 23, 1973.

Roth, D.A., Letters dated April 30, 1975, and May 7, 1975.

Roth, D.A., "She Shoots to Save," *Insight*, Washington, D.C., July 21, 1970.

Interview: Don Roth.

Chapter 31

AUSTRALIA—*Lands Down Under*

Surprise Obituary

Progress on the new Sydney Sanitarium nearly came to a halt when Dr. Daniel Kress became gravely ill only a few months after arriving from the United States. Seeing no improvement in his condition, church leaders feared the man they counted on to head their sanitarium would surely die. They appointed a time for an anointing service and asked church members to pray for him. Cables went to friends and associates in New Zealand, Tasmania, England and the United States with the brief and urgent message, "Kress is dying. Pray."

At the appointed time many prayers were offered. Within the hour the doctor began to feel better, and over the next few weeks recovered completely.

Apparently no one told his friends in the United States and England of his improved health, and soon his wife began receiving condolence letters, including one from Dr. John Harvey Kellogg of Battle Creek. Two newspapers in England published his obituary.

About three months later, a woman approached Kress at a camp meeting where he had given one of his famous health lectures.

"I thought you were dead," she said. "I am sure I read your obituary in a London paper."

The next day she brought a copy of the article headlined "The Voice We Once Heard We Shall Hear No More." In a book he wrote with his wife in 1941, Kress said he read with interest "a most delightful account" of his life and accomplishments—more than 50 years before he died!

The missionary vessel *Pitcairn* carried the first Seventh-day Adventist medical worker to the islands of the South Pacific in 1893—eight years after the first Adventist missionaries arrived in Australia. Dr. Merritt Kellogg, oldest half-brother of Dr. John Harvey Kellogg, was on the *Pitcairn's* second voyage, and for seven years worked in Tonga. Later he went to Australia to supervise construction of a sanitarium near Sydney, a facility destined to become the flagship of Adventist healthcare in the South Pacific.

Australians began traveling to Battle Creek in the late 1880s to prepare for medical missionary work. John Harvey Kellogg urged church leaders from "down under" to send him their most promising young people, warning, "We cannot make pumpkins out of small potatoes."

After these young people completed their studies, they returned to Australia inspired to begin health centers, rescue missions and other missionary work in their home country. Most of these early efforts were small and scattered, and failed for lack of money, patronage and a multitude of other problems.

About five years before plans were made for the Sydney Sanitarium, Alfred and Emma Semmens set up treatment rooms in the suburb of Ashfield. At first they recruited patients by going door-to-door. Later, with the addition of a local physician to their staff, business improved, but most patients were too poor to pay for treatments.

Some time later the couple moved into larger quarters and opened the Summer Hill Health Home. Dr. Edgar Caro joined them in 1898. Caro, an Australian who had studied at Battle Creek and Ann Arbor, Michigan, was named medical director. He provided hospital services at Summer Hill, and renamed it Medical and Surgical Sanitarium, claiming it was "more advanced than anything of its kind in Australia." He also started a nurses' training program to provide low-cost labor for the hospital and prepare medical missionaries for other areas.

Nonetheless, Summer Hill had its problems. As patronage increased, Caro rented nearby buildings that had never been intended for hospital use. Also, most of the clientele were charity cases or paid only a minimum fee. Church leaders in Australia and the South Pacific feared the inadequate setup at Summer Hill posed a high risk for patients. Ellen White, who had come to Australia in 1891, agreed that the Summer Hill facility did not "properly represent the grand and ennobling work we have to do for the Master."

So a search was begun in 1898 to find possible locations for a facility for patients who could pay for services. The Australian church leaders invited John Wessels of South Africa to manage the project, hoping he might help finance it, as he had given liberally to other healthcare and school projects. However, by the time Wessels came to Australia, the Capetown Sanitarium, which he and his family operated in South Africa, was on the brink of bankruptcy. He had no money for the Sydney project. Nonetheless, he assisted in locating a site for the new sanitarium. This led to the purchase of about 80 acres at Wahroonga on a high ridge overlooking Sydney—for only $4,200.

The Right Situation

Mrs. White traveled 80 miles from her home at Cooranbong to inspect the property. Her friend Mary Radle took her there by horse and buggy, traveling through the bush land with several others following in another cart. When Mrs. White saw the property, she said it was "a grand place—just the right situation for a sanitarium."

Drs. Daniel and Lauretta Kress joined the Summer Hill staff in 1900 after having worked earlier in England and Battle Creek. In making their travel arrangements to Sydney, they planned to spend a month in the Hawaiian Islands. However, upon arriving in Honolulu, they changed their minds and proceeded directly to Australia.

Last-minute Registration

To practice medicine in Australia, the Kresses had to register with the local medical council. Upon inquiring, they learned that the council was scheduled to meet the next day. Wasting no time, they retrieved diplomas, certificates and other important papers from their unpacked trunks and rushed them to the appropriate office to file for registration.

A secretary informed them that the council generally expected all paperwork to be on hand no less than two weeks prior to the meeting, and she could not promise that their names would be considered on such short notice. To complicate matters, only one week earlier a law had been passed ceasing recognition of American diplomas in New South Wales. In the end, the council approved the Kresses, but they were the last physicians granted a license to practice medicine in New South Wales on an American diploma. Had they spent a month in Hawaii, they likely would not have been permitted to register.

Caro had grand ideas for the new sanitarium. He envisioned a four-story brick building with 100 rooms. Much to his disappointment, church leaders put Daniel Kress in charge of building the new sanitarium, and they brought Merritt Kellogg from Tonga to design the facility and supervise construction. Kellogg drew up two plans—one along the lines of Caro's suggestions and the other a three-story timber structure. Church leaders and Mrs. White agreed to the second plan

While Caro continued to run Summer Hill, the Semmenses moved to Adelaide, and opened a treatment facility that operated for about 20 years. Others left Summer Hill and opened a health retreat at the Adventists'

Avondale School for Christian Workers at Cooranbong. It closed sometime after the new Sydney Sanitarium opened.

It was later discovered that through some questionable bookkeeping, Caro had shifted funds for the new sanitarium into the Summer Hill coffers. This all stopped in 1901 with the arrival of a new business manager—John Burden from St. Helena Sanitarium in California. Caro set up a private practice, and eventually fell out of favor with the church.

Burden instituted some cost-cutting measures and reduced the building plan to two stories with an attic. The construction crew consisted mostly of amateurs, including students from Avondale. Many worked 12 hours a day, Sunday through Thursday.

Quiet Sunday Labor

"Building on Sundays stirred some local animosity and the labourers were reported. The police visited the site on two occasions and took down their names. Police intended issuing summonses but they were not sure how they could get convictions. Kellogg reasoned with them, explaining that the sanitarium was to be for charitable work in the community. His carpenters, he added, had agreed to work fifty-seven hours per week and only accept wages for forty-eight hours. Therefore, Sunday work was their donation to a charity and they were really not earning their living by working on Sundays. Whether the argument would have survived in court will never be known for it satisfied the police and they left the workers alone. However, Kellogg took extra care to subdue noise on Sundays from that time onwards." —MILTON HOOK

Even though church leaders and members had pledged money to begin building, funds frequently ran short during construction. Nevertheless, the Lord blessed their work and the needs were always met, often at precisely the time they were most needed. Local merchants furnished lumber and other supplies on credit, and staff members did their share of fund-raising, too. One time Kellogg received wages for 18 months in a lump sum. He used part of the money to buy building materials.

Get to the Point

While Kress was attending camp meeting in Tasmania, he visited the elderly Edward Murphet, who had given generously to the church. Kress talked with him for some time, carefully avoiding the subject of money.

Finally Murphet asked him straight out, "Don't you need some money?"

Kress admitted that indeed construction was at a standstill, and yes, he needed money. Murphet ended up giving him $15,000 for the sanitarium.

Church members paid a second tithe, and special offerings were collected to keep the building program going. John Harvey Kellogg also donated royalties from the sale of his books in Australia. With only part of the building ready for patients, the sanitarium opened for business January 1, 1903. Windows were not yet installed on the third floor, and the building would not receive its first coat of paint for 10 years.

First Patient

Kellogg and others had purchased construction supplies at Lewis Butler's store in Wahroonga when they were building the sanitarium. Before it officially opened for business, Butler became ill with rheumatic fever. His family transported him by a horse-drawn cab over the rough roads to the new hospital, where he was soon on his way to recovery. While recuperating he studied the beliefs of Seventh-day Adventists and later joined the church. Many years later, his grandson, Lance Butler, was treasurer of the Australasian Division and oversaw the rebuilding of the sanitarium in the early 1970s.

When fire destroyed some of the original sanitarium in January 1919, brick was used to rebuild. Over the years the sanitarium expanded many times, usually amid voices of concern that the facility was getting extravagant. Two of the early controversies involved the installation of an X-ray machine and the addition of an elevator.

A $35 million extension in 1995 more than doubled the hospital's size. Today the 329-bed Sydney Adventist Hospital is ranked among the top 10 private hospitals in Australia. In addition to this flagship facility, at the end of the 20th century Adventists operated four other hospitals and more than 30 mission clinics in Australia, New Zealand and the islands of the South Pacific.

Victorian Home of Health

Although Mrs. White returned to the United States before the Sydney Sanitarium opened, she always remained interested in the Australia hospital. She corresponded with church leaders there and encouraged them to develop additional health centers. One of these was the Victorian

Home of Health, later called Warburton Sanitarium, established in 1910 about 50 miles from Melbourne.

The Warburton San came into being after some American missionaries vacated a house near the denomination's publishing plant. Australian church leaders converted it into a five-bed health center where two employees provided simple treatments, such as hydrotherapy, fomentations and massage. The house had piped-in water, a large bathroom, and a fireplace and one electric light fixture in each patient room. The hydroelectric plant at the publishing house supplied power.

Adventist healthcare in New Zealand began in the late 1890s and early 1900s when the church operated several little health homes and medical missions. Most of these were short-lived for lack of personnel and money. The one exception was a Health Home in Christchurch, which developed into a 10-bed sanitarium.

Pioneer missionaries Drs. Martin and Florence Keller devoted much of their time to working with the country's indigenous people, and were highly respected physicians in New Zealand. Dr. Florence was also physician to the Maori royal family.

When the Christchurch Sanitarium closed in 1921, New Zealand had no permanent Adventist hospital for more than 50 years. The church re-established its medical work in this country in 1974 by building an ultramodern facility first called New Zealand Adventist Hospital and later Auckland Adventist Hospital. The facility is now closed.

Over the years, many graduates from the various schools of nursing and other healthcare professionals traveled throughout the South Pacific islands and started clinics and dispensaries. Several hospitals, including some for sufferers of leprosy, have also operated from time to time in these islands. Today the church has two mission hospitals in the region—Sopas Adventist Hospital in Papua New Guinea, and the Atoifi Adventist Hospital in the Solomon Islands.

Big Sick Anytime

I smiled to myself when I read the signs posted at the Sopas Adventist Hospital: "Clinic Hours 8–5. Big Sick Anytime." "Fee for services 10 cents or Coconut."

I asked one of the nurses in charge of the hospital whether she was really accepting coconuts in payment for services.

"They get nothing free," she explained, directing my attention to a pile of coconuts stacked in a corner. "They can pick up a coconut on their

way to the hospital." —RAY PELTON, RETIRED ASSOCIATE DIRECTOR, HEALTH AND TEMPER-
ANCE DEPARTMENT, GENERAL CONFERENCE OF SEVENTH-DAY ADVENTISTS

SOURCES

Hook, Milton, *Hospital on a Hilltop: Pioneering the Sydney Sanitarium*, Seventh-day Adventist Heritage Series, No. 16, South Pacific Division Department of Education, undated.

Hook, Milton, *Rescue Homes and Remedies with Water: Adventist Benevolent Work in Australasia*, Seventh-day Adventist Heritage Series, No. 15, South Pacific Division Department of Education, undated.

Johns, Warren L., and Utt, Richard H., editors, *The Vision Bold,* Washington, D.C.: Review and Herald Publishing Association, 1977.

Kress, Lauretta Eby and Daniel Hartman Kress, *Under the Guiding Hand*, Washington, D.C.: College Press, 1941.

Spaulding, A. W., *Christ's Last Legion*, Washington, D.C.: Review and Herald Publishing Association, 1949.

Totenhofer, Joy, "Aunt Ellie's Husband Worked Very Hard," *Australasian Record*, October 30, 1978.

Interviews and Notes: Dr. Robert Horner and Ray Pelton.

Chapter 32

INTER-AMERICA—*Slow Growth South of the Border*

Unscheduled Surgery

Blanca Santiago had asked her friend, Blanca Pol, to go with her to Bella Vista Hospital and accompany her during surgery, a rather common practice in Puerto Rico during the 1930s and 1940s. The two women drove from San Juan to Mayaguez, where Blanca Santiago was scheduled for a thyroidectomy.

Prior to her leaving home, Blanca Pol's husband had suggested that while she was at the hospital, she should ask the doctor about an abdominal pain that had bothered her for some time. As it turned out, Blanca Santiago did not require thyroid surgery after all, but Blanca Pol needed an emergency hernia operation. The two friends went into the operating room together as planned, but in reversed roles.

Although there are more Seventh-day Adventists in Central America and the Caribbean than any other region of the world (about 2 million in 2000), the church's medical work developed slowly here. Today Adventists operate only 11 hospitals and fewer than 30 clinics throughout the region, which also includes Venezuela and Guyana in the northern part of South America. With the exception of the 150-bed Bella Vista Hospital in Puerto Rico, they range in size from only 14 to 70 beds.

The late development of Adventist healthcare in this area of the world is somewhat surprising, considering that Mexico was the first country in which the church established medical work outside the United States. Missionaries went to Guadalajara in 1893 and operated a sanitarium for a few years. After that facility closed, Adventist healthcare in Mexico consisted of only a few clinics and dispensaries, some church-sponsored, some self-supporting and some connected with local churches. These were often operated by ministers with training in simple home treatments, and most were short-lived endeavors.

Medical missionaries were also at work in other parts of Central America and the Caribbean in the late 1800s and early 1900s, and today Adventist healthcare in at least four countries traces its beginnings to these pioneers. For example, an Englishwoman who worked among the poor and sick in Jamaica went to Battle Creek for treatment. While there, she persuaded church leaders to send medical workers to that island.

On another island, an American nurse worked with the people of Trinidad from 1896 until 1905. A permanent facility, however, was not built until 1948. Also, about 1910, a sugar plantation owner from Puerto Rico was a patient at the Battle Creek Sanitarium, and thereafter hired an Adventist doctor to care for his employees.

There is little doubt that the people of Central America and the Caribbean needed healthcare services, but several factors delayed building permanent facilities.

While there may not have been a lack of patients, there was a shortage of people willing to replace the missionaries who died or returned to their homeland. For one thing, some countries required physicians to take a rigid examination in Spanish, and some countries simply did not put out a welcome mat for foreign missionaries. Missionaries were robbed, some were murdered, and some suffered or died of typhoid, yellow fever, malaria and other tropical diseases. Scarcity of proper food and housing, shortage of funds, political revolutions, superstition, hurricanes, earthquakes and many other problems sent discouraged missionaries back to the United States. In writing about early attempts to establish medical work in Mexico City, Wesley Amundsen seems to have accurately described the climate in which early missionaries labored in Central America, when he said, "the winds of adversity blew cold."

While their medical work may have had a slow beginning, Adventist missionaries continued to preach the gospel and establish schools wherever they could. All of the earliest attempts at clinics and sanitariums eventually closed. Most of today's hospitals in Central America and the Caribbean opened after 1960. Exceptions are Montemorelos University Hospital in Mexico, Andrews Memorial Hospital in Jamaica, Davis Memorial Clinic and Hospital in Guyana and Bella Vista Hospital in Puerto Rico.

Mexico's 63-bed Montemorelos University Hospital started as a clinic connected with a local church. In the 1940s the clinic moved to a new hospital built on donated land near an Adventist college. Today's Montemorelos University Hospital provides clinical training for medical students, nurses and other healthcare professionals.

Jamaica also built a permanent hospital in the 1940s, and named it in honor of the first Seventh-day Adventist overseas missionary, John Nevins Andrews. Andrews Memorial Hospital opened in 1946, thanks in part to support from the College of Medical Evangelists in Loma Linda, California.

Adventists started medical work in Guyana in the 1950s, first in a small clinic built with materials from a U.S. airbase, and then a hospital in 1955. It was a simple building with no running water. Because the lights had not been installed in time for the first surgery, the mission president assisted the doctor by holding a desk lamp over the patient. A replacement facility built in the mid-1960s was named in honor of Ovid Davis, missionary to Guyana who died of malaria while working with the Arecuna and Akawai Indians in the early 1900s.

Other Adventist hospitals in Central America and the Caribbean in 2000 include Adventist Hospital of Haiti, Antillean Adventist Hospital in Netherlands Antilles, Cave Memorial Clinic and Nursing Home in Barbados, Southeast Hospital in Mexico, Valley of the Angels Hospital in Honduras and Venezuela Adventist Hospital in Venezuela.

SOURCE

Amundson, Wesley, *The Advent Message in Inter-America*, Washington, D.C.: Review and Herald Publishing Association, 1947.

Chapter 33

INTER-AMERICA—*Sweet Beginnings in Puerto Rico*

Hot Ride to Ensenada

The train had no air-conditioning and the weather was so hot William and Hattie Dunscombe opened some windows, letting in dozens of mosquitoes. Mrs. Dunscombe worried all night that the children might fall from their bunks and through the windows. The 110-mile trip finally ended at Ensenada.

Adventist medical work in Puerto Rico began in a sugar plantation around 1910, soon after Mr. Grief, the plantation manager, went to Battle Creek to recuperate from "nervous exhaustion." While staying there, he decided to hire a Seventh-day Adventist physician for the plantation. The first two stayed only a short time. Finally Dr. John Morse arrived in 1912. He was the plantation physician for eight years, and during this time generously supported the Seventh-day Adventist Church in Puerto Rico.

Learning of the need for doctors on the island, Dr. William Dunscombe went to Puerto Rico in 1920. He had previously worked in South Africa, Japan and the Wabash Sanitarium in Indiana.

The Dunscombes' first house had no window screens. Due to the threat of malaria, the children studied under mosquito netting and the family usually retired to their mosquito-net-covered beds right after supper. Malaria seemed to strike most everyone, complicating other diseases, as well as surgical and obstetrical cases.

Except during the three years he worked at New England Sanitarium and Hospital in Massachusetts, Dunscombe remained in Puerto Rico for 40 years. His used to walk or use a horse and buggy to make house calls as he cared for several thousand agricultural laborers on the plantation.

Helping Hand

In those days, factory and field workers received about 70 cents for a 12-hour workday, and the fieldwork lasted only six months a year. A true missionary at heart, Dunscombe helped establish a feeding program, bringing in truckloads of bananas, rice, beans and other staples to the workers and their large families.

~

The sugar company allowed Dunscombe to operate a private practice, which was very successful. He used the income from this work to build churches in Puerto Rico, and dreamed of one day opening a hospital, too. That dream was realized when he learned that a hospital in Mayaguez, about 30 miles from Ensenada, was for sale. He bought it at a fraction of its value and soon two other physicians joined him—his son Dr. Colby Dunscombe, who had completed a residency in eye, ear, nose and throat at White Memorial Hospital in Los Angeles, and Dr. Charles Moore, who helped with surgery and general practice.

Dunscombe then bought a clinic in 1941 and opened what was known as the Dunscombe Hospital. Though the government took over this facility during World War II, he received enough money to purchase a large house, which he remodeled and opened as the Polyclinic Bella Vista. It was a very popular endeavor, attracting patients from all over the island. Eventually the doctors entered into an arrangement with the Seventh-day Adventist Church whereby they accepted denominational-level wages and donated the earnings from their medical practices to establish a permanent hospital.

By 1947 plans were underway to raise $75,000 for a 20-bed hospital. It soon grew to 80 beds thanks in part to U.S. funding available through the Hill-Burton Act of 1946. As the size of the project grew, the cost jumped to $600,000, greatly straining the church's resources. Although construction began in February 1951, it stopped at the end of the year when the architect broke his contract. The sounds of construction resumed in April 1952, only to be interrupted a few months later when the contractor defaulted. Finally A.L. Christensen, a builder at the Adventists' Antillean College in Cuba, finished the hospital. The new Bella Vista Hospital opened January 4, 1954.

During this time Christensen's daughter, Elaine, was a secretary at the denomination's Inter-American Division office in Coral Gables, Florida. In an interesting turn of events, one year after the hospital opened, her new husband, Royce Thompson, became administrator of the new hospital; they served there for 13 years.

SOURCES

Interviews and Notes: Margaret Donaldson, wife of Bella Vista Hospital physician, provided unpublished manuscripts written by Hattie Dunscombe, Phyllis Dunscombe and Beulah Christensen, written about

1964. Hattie Dunscombe was wife of Dr. William Dunscombe; Phyllis Dunscombe was their daughter-in-law and a nursing instructor; and Beulah Christensen, wife of A.L. Christensen, was a schoolteacher.

Chapter 34

EUROPE—Bathtubs, Elastics and A King's Villa

Apostle of Health

The Skodsborg Sanitarium near Copenhagen was at one time the largest health institution in Scandinavia and one of Europe's largest. Founder and director, Dr. J.C. Ottosen, pioneered physiotherapy in Scandinavia. He established a health-food factory, as well as schools of physical therapy, nursing and dietetics, whose graduates served all over the world. The king of Denmark knighted Ottosen for his contribution to health and temperance. When the doctor died in 1942, newspapers throughout Scandinavia referred to him as the "Health Apostle of the North."

Danish-born Ottosen, who had operated a clinic at Frydenstrand for a short time in the late 1890s, found a beautifully developed property fit for a king near Copenhagen. In fact, it had been a resort for Danish royalty for many years. When Ottosen found this "King's Villa," it was in the hands of Christian IX, an elderly widower whose children had grown and left home. Having no use for the property, he sold it to the Adventist church, and Ottosen converted it into a 20-bed sanitarium. The impressive Skodsborg Sanitarium, sometimes called "The White Village," eventually grew to nearly 300 beds. It was located on a busy highway used for many years by thousands of tourists visiting the Kronborg Castle.

Skodsborg operated a sanitarium-style program longer than any other Adventist healthcare organization, and served as a model for nearly a dozen similar facilities in northern Europe. Throughout its 94-year history, people came here for hydrotherapy, massage, therapeutic baths and exercise activities ranging from badminton to horseback riding and swimming. Health-minded guests always had a wide choice of dishes from the dining room's bountiful smorgasbord, including items from the church's Danish food factory. Musical programs and health lectures rounded out the sanitarium program.

Skodsborg operated without disruption, except when Germany took it over in World War II. During that time the physicians and staff cared for German soldiers.

In later years, a lifestyle center and a heart-rehabilitation program were added, but Skodsborg never offered services associated with a general acute-care hospital. These were provided by Denmark's state medical program. Much of the sanitarium's success was attributed to a large subsidy by the city of Copenhagen for government employees' use of the facility. Loss of that contract, combined with the failure of the food company and other factors, led to the closure of Skodsborg Sanitarium in 1992.

Health education, physiotherapy, hydrotherapy and rehabilitation have been the hallmarks of Adventist healthcare in Europe for more than a century. Because many European countries have national health programs, most Adventist facilities in this part of the world have retained the health resort nature of the early sanitariums.

As in other parts of the world, the European health ventures that started around the turn of the 20th century had close ties to the Battle Creek Sanitarium. From humble beginnings in the late 1800s and early 1900s, today the church operates eight hospitals and health centers in Europe, in addition to many retirement homes and nursing homes. Schools of nursing and physical therapy associated with these centers have graduated hundreds of healthcare professionals who have contributed to the growth and mission of the church's worldwide medical ministry.

Adventist Healthcare Swiss Style

The pioneer doctor who established the first Adventist health center in Switzerland was never legally the physician in charge because he did not have a Swiss diploma. Canadian-born Dr. Perry DeForest opened a health institute, school of nursing, and food factory in Basel around 1895. After about 10 years he moved his work to the present location of the Lake Geneva Sanitarium at Gland, where he directed its activities until he retired in 1935. The hospital gradually expanded over the years and now houses 92 patient beds.

☙

Drs. Daniel and Lauretta Kress of Battle Creek arrived in England in 1899 to establish Adventist medical work in Great Britain, only to discover no money was available for treatment rooms or a sanitarium. Not losing sight of the need to eventually establish a health center, the innovative pioneers started giving health lectures and began a health magazine.

Uncovering Dress Reform

"At that time the women of England were wearing very tight corsets, and all their clothes were hung from the hips. I had on a union suit, and

elastics that hung from my shoulders. They were pretty, being made of pink silk, with pink elastic that would give when I bent over. I had on only two other garments, a slip that hung from my shoulders and a dress which did the same. I had devised a lining in my dress which gave me plenty of room for expansion if I wished to exercise in the dress. I began talking about this lining, and said, 'I can better demonstrate it by showing my dress that I have on.' At that I loosened it at the shoulders and laid back the front, which showed the lining.

"The ladies wanted a nearer view of it, and asked if I would not take off my dress so they might see it. There was a large assembly of women present. A lady came forward and got my dress, and I did not see it again for about an hour. They asked to see my slip, and I took it off also, and stood lecturing to that crowd of women in conservative England in my under suit and pink elastics." —DR. LAURETTA KRESS

∼

Finally church leaders began thinking seriously about starting a sanitarium in England. The first place they showed the Kresses was in a poor section of London where area residents could not afford to pay for services. Seeing there was no room for expansion, and people from other areas would not be inclined to travel into the area for medical care, the doctors rejected the location.

About a week later a letter arrived from Ellen White, assuring the Kresses they had made the right choice in turning down the first proposed site. She counseled them to find a place at least 20 miles from London, "where the air was not contaminated with smoke and dust." It was not long before they found just such a place—a former women's college, complete with a vegetable garden, flower garden, tennis court and place to play croquet. A spacious building provided plenty of room for staff and patents.

"We felt God had indeed led us to this lovely spot," Dr. Lauretta said.

When it came to furnishing the sanitarium, a wealthy man who had attended some of their lectures donated the entire contents of his home—everything from a piano to linens and china.

The Kresses' stay in England ended prematurely and tragically when their oldest daughter died. Although they would have continued their term in Great Britain, Dr. Daniel suffered from the climate and overwork. Attempting to restore his health, he spent one winter in France, but finally returned to the United States, leaving his wife to carry on the sanitarium work in England. She later joined him in the United States, where they remained until 1900 when they went to Australia.

Stanboroughs of England

Adventists operated a number of small sanitariums in Great Britain in the early 1900s, but eventually all the healthcare work was merged into the Stanborough Park Sanitarium in England. "The Stanboroughs" as it was nicknamed, operated continuously from 1912 to 1968. Plans to enlarge the facility in the 1940s never materialized because the government used it during World War II. By the time it was returned to the church, England had a national health plan. When The Stanboroughs closed, all nursing services were transferred to Crieff, Scotland, where Dr. Gertrude Brown operated the forerunner of today's Roundelwood Good Health Association.

Brown had studied nursing at the sanitarium in Switzerland. She then worked in Ireland, where she met and married Dr. Edward Brown. They eventually settled in Scotland and opened the Crieff Nursing Home.

After her husband died, Dr. Gertrude sold the facility to the church in 1966 with the request that it be operated on the Battle Creek model. A dynamic public speaker in high demand for health lectures, she served as Roundelwood's medical supervisor until her death in 1974 at age 95. Today the 51-bed facility offers such services as physiotherapy, hydrotherapy, occupational therapy, a gymnasium and toning salon.

Early Adventist healthcare in Germany may have somewhat resembled today's home-health services. The church started a school of nursing in connection with a sanitarium in Friedensau in the early 1900s. Graduates of this program lived in homes established throughout Germany and worked in private-duty care. At one time 52 nurses were working from 18 of these homes. Two other important centers for early Adventist medical work in Germany were Berlin and Wiesbaden.

Today's 230-bed Berlin Hospital opened in 1920 as the 39-bed Waldfriede Sanitarium and Clinic. This hospital has operated a school of nursing since 1923, and also offers internship and residency programs.

In Sweden Adventists have operated health centers ever since the Nyhyttan Health and Rehabilitation Center opened as a summer health resort in 1905. Nyhyttan offered a vegetarian diet and hydrotherapy treatments given in old wooden bathtubs. From 1933 until it closed in 1997, Nyhyttan operated year-round, providing hydrotherapy, as well as physiotherapy and rehabilitation services.

Today in Sweden Adventists operate Hultafors Health Centre, established in 1927. This facility specializing in hydrotherapy, dietetics and rehabilitation is located on 365 acres on a wooded mountain ridge. The beautiful eight-story center features an indoor swimming pool on the top floor, overlooking Lake Viaredsjon and a forest below. Hultafors has never offered general hospital services. Most patients come for physiotherapy or cardiovascular problems. In addition, the center runs a small program for drug and alcohol rehabilitation. Some guests continue to come for rest and restoration.

A similar center in Finland opened in the 1920s and continues operation today. The original Hydro-Electric Institute shared a building with local church headquarters from 1926 until 1943 when land was purchased for the Hopeaniema Sanitarium. Located about 30 miles from Helsinki, this was the first year-round Adventist-owned sanitarium in Finland.

The North Norway Rehabilitation Center, located above the Arctic Circle at Tromoso, has the distinction of being the northernmost Adventist healthcare facility. Established in 1952, it is one of two health centers the church operates in Norway. The other is the 150-bed Skogli Health and Rehabilitation Center in Lillehammer, established in 1946. Although each of these facilities opened about 50 years ago, two Battle Creek graduates operating a clinic in Oslo actually started the first Adventist medical work in Norway more than 100 years ago. The health programs in Norway have always focused on physiotherapy and rehabilitation.

SOURCES

Kress, Lauretta Eby and Daniel Hartman Kress, *Under the Guiding Hand*, Washington, D.C.: College Press, 1941.

"Denmark Sanitarium Forced to Close," *Adventist Review*, July 30, 1992.

Hartmann, Walder, "Sanitarium Develops from Royal Residence into Modern Health Resort," *Adventist Review*, April 27, 1989.

du Chemin, Audrey, "The White Village," *Loma Linda University Alumni Journal*, September 1967.

Interviews: Mazie Herin, Ray Pelton and Alice Smith.

Chapter 35

SOUTH AMERICA— From Argentina to the Amazon
Mission Assignment

"Although we were officially missionaries, we saw at once the diseases rampant on the Amazon and we knew that we had first to concentrate on making these people well.... We had not come to impose by force or fear our ideas or culture or dogmas; we had come to help other human beings. This was our assignment." —LEO B. HALLIWELL

Efforts by early missionaries who endured extreme hardships, religious opposition and political instability laid the groundwork for what would eventually become a strong network of Adventist hospitals in South America. Today the church operates more than 20 hospitals and clinics and a dozen medical launches on this continent.

Much of the first mission endeavors focused on education and church growth, but all missionaries needed some knowledge of basic healthcare. Many of them suffered, and some died from tropical diseases. Poor transportation, usually by horse and over treacherous mountain trails, greatly hindered their work. Often the challenges were beyond their training. For example, when Orley Ford went to Peru in 1917, an Indian asked him to treat his son's foot. Gangrene had already spread to the knee. With only four months of training in "medical techniques" and no surgical equipment, the missionary amputated the leg using a butcher knife and saw. The patient survived, and Ford later made him a wooden leg.

It took a certain kind of person to be a missionary in those days, and South America had some of the best. Among the most well known were Ferdinand and Ana Stahl in Peru and Bolivia, Robert and Della Habenicht in Argentina, and Leo and Jessie Halliwell in Brazil. The efforts of these pioneers, as well as many others, to relieve human suffering in South America went a long way in creating goodwill and breaking through walls of misunderstanding.

Few towns in Argentina had physicians—let alone hospitals or clinics—in 1901, when the Habenichts arrived at the mission at Puiggari (now Libartodor San Martin), Entre Rios. At first the doctor-nurse team from Iowa traveled in horse-drawn wagons over very poor roads to care for patients in rural areas. They set up a clinic in their mission home, where they did everything from simple hydrotherapy treatments to surgery. When patients needed a bed, their children and the nurses who assisted with the medical work gave up their beds. Up to 20 patients stayed in the house at one time.

Eventually plans came together to build a small hospital. Church members donated land, materials and labor, and true to their missionary spirit, the Habenichts gave liberally to the project. The one-story, six-bed River Plate Sanitarium and Hospital opened in 1908.

The Habenichts' personal sacrifice to relieve human suffering went a long way in creating goodwill, but in the early days the doctor and the church had their enemies, too. One neighbor tried to kill Habenicht. Another, hoping to close the hospital, started a rumor that the doctor had died. In time, of course, people learned to trust the Habenichts, and appreciated their 21 years of service at River Plate.

Dr. Charles Westphal took over leadership of the hospital in 1923. The son of the first Adventist minister in South America, Westphal had lived in Argentina since he was four years old. He served at River Plate Sanitarium and Hospital for 35 years.

Because of its remote location and lack of population base, the hospital did not grow for many years. Tito Weiss, former chief financial officer of Adventist Health System and now retired in Florida, grew up in Crespo, near the River Plate community, and worked at the hospital in the late 1950s. In fact, his grandfather was involved in developing both the hospital and River Plate College. Weiss says when he was young there was nothing in the area except the school and hospital and a beautiful view.

For many years the only means of transportation to Puiggari was horse and buggy. Undeveloped roads and rivers prone to flooding during the rainy season made traveling difficult, if not impossible. Weiss recalls a 10-mile stretch of road where cars often got stuck when it rained. Since the town had no hotels, local residents opened their homes to visitors stuck in Puiggari.

Things began to improve about the mid-1930s with the construction of a bridge. This helped draw patients to the sanitarium, some traveling up to 200 miles for simple outpatient procedures or physical examinations. In addition, local residents began opening hotels and restaurants to accommodate visitors.

The hospital's financial turnaround came during the 1950s and 1960s, under the direction of Dr. Marcelo Hammerly, who had been with the hospital since 1937. Also three graduates of River Plate College—Pedro Tabuenca, Dario Rostan and Arturo Weiss—returned to the sanitarium after completing medical studies at Argentinean universities. Gradually business increased as people heard about the excellent care and services provided by these doctors and the sanitarium staff. Clients continued to travel great distances to enjoy the benefits of hydrotherapy, massage and other treatments.

In addition to a growing medical staff, development of the college to university status with a school of medicine also contributed to the sanitarium's growth. River Plate University School of Health Sciences is the second Adventist medical school for Spanish-speaking students. The first is in Montemorelos, Mexico.

As River Plate became firmly established, it was possible for some of the staff to begin hospitals elsewhere in South America. One of these was a 42-bed facility in an affluent neighborhood of Buenos Aires, where some of the residential mansions stretch for an entire block. After the church's South American headquarters moved from this community to Uruguay in the 1950s, physicians converted the building into Belgrano Adventist Medical Clinic.

The 43-bed Loma Linda Adventist Sanitarium opened in 1966 in response to the request of River Plate patients who wished to have a similar facility in north Argentina. Dr. Juan Carlos Moroni joined Dr. Weiss to open a clinic at Presidencia Roque Saenz Pena, and within a year, plans were laid for a sanitarium.

The youngest Adventist healthcare facility in Argentina is also second largest. The 50-bed Northeast Argentine Sanitarium was established in 1972.

In Paraguay, three graduate nurses from River Plate Sanitarium and Hospital opened a small physiotherapy clinic in 1945. Then with the arrival of Dr. Ira E. Bailie, a Loma Linda University graduate, plans were soon underway to build a hospital. The Paraguay Sanitarium and Hospital, later renamed Asuncion Adventist Sanitarium, was immediately successful and soon outgrew the original facility. The hospital has been enlarged and modernized several times over the years.

Some time after the Asuncion sanitarium opened, residents near the Argentina border raised funds and built the Hohenau Adventist Sanitarium and Hospital in 1965. Medical staff from Asuncion and Argentina provided medical staff coverage.

The names of Ferdinand and Ana Stahl are synonymous with early Adventist missions in Peru and Bolivia. After studying nursing and then operating treatment rooms in Ohio for a brief time, the young Stahls volunteered for service to South America in 1909. For the next 29 years they established missions, schools and clinics in Peru and Bolivia.

Strong People

"There once came to us a chief from a distant region, who had had his middle finger torn off, it having become entangled in a rope attached to an ox that became frightened. In his crude way, he had tried to cure the finger by tying over it a piece of sheep's liver. When he came to us, over a month afterward, his hand had become badly infected.... We had no anaesthetic on hand at that time; and I explained to the man what would have to be done in order to save his hand, if not his life. I told him that it was going to hurt, but that we would not hurt him any more than was positively necessary. While talking to him, I put my arm around him; and when I had finished explaining to him, he put out his injured hand to me, and said, 'Father, you can go right ahead and do what you think is best.' Then, taking from his head a woolen cap such as the Indians in that region always wear, he crowded it into his mouth as far as possible. I asked my interpreter what the man meant by this. 'Oh,' he said, 'he is stuffing his mouth full so that he will not cry out and will have something to bite on!' I removed the finger at the last joint, cut away the putrid flesh, applied the antiseptics, and bandaged the stump. The man never flinched." —F.A. STAHL

Wherever the Stahls went, people came to them for medical care. In his book, *In the Land of the Incas*, Stahl said that news of their arrival usually spread like wildfire, as the following selections illustrate.

Confident Patients

"When we arrived at the distant places to which we had been called, we would find the people gathered by hundreds with their sick to be treated. Whole provinces were down with smallpox and typhoid fever.

"At the same time that we were caring for the people, we carried on an educational campaign among them, teaching them how to keep well. We vaccinated many, thus staying the spread of smallpox."

"We had to do considerable minor surgery, and the confidence the Indians put in us was really wonderful. They thought we were able to do almost everything. Many a one has come to us, telling us that he had pains in his chest, and asking if we would not please cut out his lungs and heart. At other times, some would ask for memory medicine, or for some medicine to make them good."

The Stahls pulled teeth, performed surgery, gave smallpox vaccinations, cleaned filthy water springs that caused typhoid epidemics, administered fomentations and compresses in fever cases, and taught the Indians to use water inside and out to stave off disease.

"We found that cleanliness, with plenty of pure water to drink, and the simplest treatments, worked marvels," said Stahl.

Seeing is Believing

"Many times, the people did not wholly follow our instructions in reference to drinking pure water and using the simple compresses and fomentations, because it was difficult for them to believe that clear water would be a help to them. So we would leave with them a coloring matter to put into the water; and after that, they would follow directions implicitly, applying compresses as instructed."

Today Adventists operate three hospitals in Peru. The oldest, Juliaca Adventist Clinic, opened in 1922 in a rented house. Dr. S. Theron Johnston secured contracts to provide healthcare for a major railway system and various government organizations, which eventually comprised about half of the clinic's business. In 1946 the church acquired a former German embassy residence in Lima and opened Good Hope Clinic, the predecessor of today's 90-bed Miraflores Adventist Clinic. The Ana Stahl Adventist Clinic, named in honor of the pioneer missionary, opened in 1961 under the direction of a Dr. Rodolfo, who in recent years has initiated a public health program for jungle villages.

Bolivia has two small Adventist medical facilities today, the 14-bed La Paz Adventist Clinic and the East Bolivia Adventist Clinic with eight beds. However, for many years the church's medical work in Bolivia was pretty much a hit-or-miss situation. During the Stahls' brief stay from 1909 to 1911, they provided health services to the affluent population in La Paz, and later worked among the Indians. Although the local mission tried to continue the medical work after they left, religious opposition, persecution and tropical diseases greatly hindered their efforts.

Finally things began to improve in 1929 with the arrival of Dr. H.E. Butka, whose work helped change negative attitudes. The local government built a hospital for Butka in 1931, calling it Hospital Adventista Chulumani. The church operated it until about 1970.

Opportunity came in 1946 to operate another Bolivian hospital—Guayaramerin Hospital on the Madera River. Dr. Harry Pitman, who served as medical director of both Chulumani and Guayaramerin, bought two war surplus airplanes to travel between the hospitals. Unfortunately, one plane crashed into a mountainside, killing the doctor and pilot. Adventists operated Guayaramerin off and on until 1967.

After four years in Peru, Orley and Lillian Ford were asked to begin a mission at Colta in 1921 to work among the Indians in the highlands of Ecuador. They arrived during a drought, and soon found themselves being blamed for the lack of rain. It got so bad that the Fords knew if it did not rain, they had no chance of working among these people. They called a prayer meeting, which attracted about 50 brave Indians who expected a sign of God's displeasure.

"They sat there with bowed heads, afraid to look each other in the face; yet they felt that this had to be risked in order to save their crops," said Mrs. Ford.

That very night it began to rain. In fact, it kept raining until people began thinking they might have to ask the missionaries to stop the rain. This experience brought a turning point in the Fords' mission to Ecuador.

Flooded with Patients

"Soon crowds were coming to our little hut to receive relief from their many ills. We were so busy that we hardly had time to eat. At five o'clock in the morning the yard would be filled with waiting sick. Our one room served as private home, hospital, and clinic. The dining table served as operating table, where all sorts of minor surgery were done. Our stack of kerosene boxes piled one on top of the other was our drug store to which people came from far and near to buy their common remedies. A large stone just outside our door served as dental chair where teeth were extracted, cleaned, or treated." —LILLIAN FORD

Despite repeated setbacks Adventist medical work finally got started in Ecuador in the 1950s. Dr. Waldo W. Stiles established a successful private practice in Quito in 1957. He even built a hospital, which he and his wife donated to the church in 1961. In addition to inpatient services, today the 21-bed Quito Adventist Clinic operates a dispensary that provides free care to thousands of people every year.

The early days of Adventist medical work in Brazil bring to mind images of mission launches plying the waters of the Amazon with doctors and nurses dispensing medicines, treating injuries, distributing food and clothing and preaching the gospel in remote areas of the country. Leo and Jessie Halliwell, missionaries in Brazil from 1921 to 1959, started this unique outreach in 1931.

Until that time the church's medical work in Brazil was limited, even though missionaries began coming here in the late 1800s. Seeing the needs of the people living along some 40,000 miles of Amazon waterways stretching between Belem and Manaus, Halliwell came up with the idea of a specially designed boat for one of the world's largest rivers. The church's youth in the United States raised more than $5,000 to build the first of these vessels, called *Luzeiro*, meaning "bearer of light." Halliwell, a trained engineer, designed and constructed it by hand—without a circular saw, power saw or planer. In *Light in the Jungle*, he describes his strange-looking craft.

An Unusual Vessel

"The boat I designed was thirty-three feet long, ten feet wide, and drew only two and a half feet of water. It had a double-V bottom—the two V's ran the length of the boat, one on each side, with a space between. The bottom was designed in a convex curve slightly higher at the center keel than at the edges. This gave us a little dead space under the boat that helped to keep the boat steady. The double V was useful in many ways. The boat would stand safely on its V-shaped haunches when the tide ran out, and this gave us an easy method of cleaning the bottom or making emergency repairs on a mud flat miles from civilization.

"Once the boat was on paper, I had to have materials and a place to build. I found a yard in Belem...but the man who owned it was dismayed at my design, told me it was unlike anything he had ever heard of, and said it would turn over the moment it hit the water. He finally agreed to let me build it in his yard but only on the condition that I would not hold him responsible for the disaster he was certain would come with the launching....

"At last the boat was finished. She was a strange-looking craft, I had to admit, more like a houseboat than a river-going launch. Yet she was sleek and slim, bright and sparkling, with her white paint and gray-and-black trim....

"July 4, 1931—approximately three months after we had begun to search for wood—the Luzeiro was launched. Jessie christened her with a bottle of imitation champagne that was simply soda water while forty of our church people watched. The Luzeiro slid down the ways and floated nicely—exactly at the line that I had marked as the center of buoyancy.

"The first man on board was the boatyard owner, effusive with his excited congratulations." —LEO HALLIWELL

❧

177

One mission launch eventually grew into a fleet of several boats, which Halliwell supervised for many years. As the Amazon work became well-known, pharmaceutical companies and government agencies provided medicines and supplies. For 30 years the Halliwells traveled the great winding river, caring for a quarter of a million people and preaching the gospel, as illustrated in the following segment from *Light in the Jungle*.

Familiar Call

A young boy approached the boat. "'Mister, have you any medicine for the fever?'" he asked.

It was a question Leo and Jessie Halliwell would hear thousands of times as they traveled the Amazon. The boy explained that several people up the river were sick. The Halliwells assured him they would help.

"I will never forget the sight that greeted us as we went into his house. The roof and walls were of thatched palm leaves, held up by poles on the sides and with one main support in the middle of the one large room. From that center post, radiating out to the side walls like spokes of some giant, quivering wheel, were twenty-one hammocks, and in each of these was someone who was sick.

"Some were shaking with the malaria chills. Others were burning with high fever, motionless and gaunt. Still others had broken out into a cold sweat. At that time all we had with us to treat this disease was quinine; more specific drugs and treatments were to come years later. But quinine we had. We sterilized our needles and began to inject it. It was obvious that the treatment did good, not only medically but psychologically; some one was doing something; these people were not merely being left there to die."

While the mission launch program has grown in recent years, today the Adventist church in Brazil also operates nine modern hospitals, in addition to several clinics and dispensaries. Two of these hospitals—Belem Adventist Hospital, 110 beds, established in 1953, and Manaus Adventist Hospital, 50 beds, established in1978—are located in cities on either end of the Amazon, where the Halliwells often visited.

The church's oldest hospital in Brazil is the 40-bed Sao Paulo Adventist Hospital, founded in 1942. With 140 patient beds, the largest is Silvestre Adventist Hospital in Rio de Janeiro, established in 1948. The 13-bed Espirito Santo Adventist Hospital, established in 1982, is the smallest, and the newest is the 60-bed Nova Friburgo Adventist Hospital, which opened in 1997. The remaining three include Sao Roque Adventist Clinic, 50 beds, established in 1980; Porto Alegre Adventist Clinic, an outpatient hospital established in1989; and Penfigo Adventist Hospital, 104 beds, opened in 1950.

Interestingly, Penfigo Adventist Hospital was established after a minister discovered a treatment for an endemic skin disease commonly known as *fogo selvagem* also called "savage fire" or "wildfire." Don Christman recorded the experience in his book, *Savage Fire.*

Cure for Savage Disease

Barbosa de Souze's wife lay on death's doorstep, her body covered with painful blisters. After months of dead-end leads, his search led him to a train station where he saw a woman with strange black skin. Impulsively he approached the man accompanying her.

"She had fogo selvagem, *but is cured now," the man said.*

Alfredo could hardly believe it. Then the stranger told him about a man named Isidoro Jamar, a trained pharmacist near the Paraguay border. Jamar, who had become a reclusive alcoholic, had developed a pitch-based salve containing linseed oil and something he called a "body-fortifying" medicine. It was a highly toxic concoction that he initially tested on a cat. While the treatment sent the animal screeching into the jungle, it later returned completely healed. After that, Jamar used it for savage fire.

Alfredo traveled to Jamar's village only to find him so drunk he had to wait several hours for him to sober up. Jamar wanted Alfredo to bring his wife to him for treatment, but Alfredo was sure she could not endure the trip. He finally persuaded Jamar to teach him how to apply the medicine.

The next morning, after bathing his wife with a "brew" made of eucalyptus branches to anesthetize her body, Alfredo applied the pitch-based ointment. Within minutes Aurea was screaming for her life—throwing herself onto her bed and then to the floor. She said it was as though a red-hot torch had been set to her whole body. But after a second treament, she was cured.

Word of her healing spread quickly and soon others were coming to Alfredo for help. By March 1949 so many people were seeking treatment that the mission set up a special program. This effort eventually developed into the Penfigo Adventist Hospital. In the first dozen years, the staff provided free care for more than 600 sufferers of fogo selvagem. Around 1960 a Dr. Gunter Hans worked with some pharmacists to make an improved, less toxic salve.

SOURCES

Christman, Don R., *Savage Fire*, Washington, D.C.: Review and Herald Publishing Association, 1961.

Ford, Mrs. Orley, *In the High Andes*, Nashville, Tennessee: Southern Publishing Association, 1932.

Halliwell, Leo B., *Light in the Jungle*, Mountain View, California: Pacific Press Publishing Association, 1959.

Stahl, F. A., *In the Land of the Incas*, Mountain View, California: Pacific Press Publishing Association, 1920.

SDA Document File 3541.19, Del Webb Library, Heritage Room, Loma Linda University, Loma Linda, California.

Interview: Tito Weiss.

Part 3

Post-World War II

Chapter 36

Bucket Brigades, Quilt Raffles and Multi-million-dollar Gifts

Times of Change

Post-World War II brought a new era of Adventist healthcare in the United States. The driving force was quite different from the early years when the focus was primarily on finding suitable locations, where people could benefit from fresh air, outdoor activities and a relaxing environment. While the sanitariums offered medical and surgical services, many patients traveled long distances to spend several weeks in a sanitarium's health-resort environment. This changed after World War II.

The post-war years brought many advances such as new vaccines, antibiotics, technologies and know-how. They also brought insurance, Medicare and government regulations. Adventist sanitariums saw a decline in traditional business, while acute-care business accelerated. Patient stays dropped from months to days. The post-war years also brought government funding, thanks to the Hill-Burton Act and other programs. Communities began to look at their own healthcare needs, and many turned to the Seventh-day Adventist Church for help.

With more than 80 years of experience, Adventists had a reputation for managing hospitals around the world. Additionally, their schools were producing physicians, nurses and other professionals to establish and staff healthcare facilities.

Many communities in the United States had no hospital, requiring residents to travel several miles for healthcare services, or do without. In other places hospitals had closed for various reasons and communities wanted to reopen them. There were also a few communities in which physicians had established small facilities and then gave them to the church. In addition, some philanthropic-minded individuals gave money to build hospitals to honor their parents.

Changes in healthcare reimbursement and insurance in the 1980s and 1990s mandated that hospitals unite in strong organizations in order to obtain insurance contracts, streamline management and benefit from economies of scale. This involved a variety of arrangements from outright gifts to the church to management leases of community-owned facilities. All Adventist-operated hospitals established after World War II represented the combined effort of local communities and the church or its health systems.

As the genesis of the post-World War II hospitals varied, so did the means to fund them. Millions of dollars for these community hospitals came from philanthropists, foundations, corporations and government organizations. Without a doubt, some of the most interesting fund-raising experiences involved soliciting community support. These are stories of quilt sales, pocket change collected in plastic buckets, and dollar bills stuffed into mailing tubes or crumpled paper bags. As the stories reveal, people put their hearts and souls into these hospitals, often working for little or no salary. At the same time, there are stories of abundant blessings.

The story of North York Branson Hospital is included in this section because it was the only large community hospital Adventists ever operated in Canada. Like its sister hospitals in the United States, Branson represented the combined efforts of a local community and the church.

Chapter 37

Resort Reborn

Florida Hospital Heartland Medical Center
Established 1948

It's All Yours

Marvyn Baldwin could not believe his eyes as he stood before the open warehouse door. It was full of equipment and furnishings from a World War II hospital ship—everything from beds and operating tables to sterilizers, chairs and mattresses.

"It's all yours," the government official said.

Then Baldwin could hardly believe his ears when the man told him, "You've got two days to get it out of here."

Baldwin got a truck and crew and started hauling loads to Avon Park. They emptied the warehouse within the two-day limit and a few weeks later opened the doors of an old hotel that had been converted into a 63-bed hospital.

Originally known as Walker Memorial Sanitarium and Hospital, today's Florida Hospital Heartland Medical Center traces its roots to an abandoned facility, which at various times housed a resort, health center, hotel, casino and military training center. Adventists converted it into a hospital in 1948.

In 1925 someone built a large hotel on the shores of Lake Lillian (known then as Highlands Lake), which attracted many vacationers seeking Florida's warm winter weather. Business was so good that the owners added a casino and 18-hole golf course. However, after the stock market crash of 1929, business declined and the place went bankrupt. The huge hotel and casino remained vacant until a woman named Helen Randle purchased it in 1936.

Claiming to be a doctor, Randle convinced Avon Park residents to invest in what she promised would be an innovative health-and-fitness center. After raising money for the project, she left town, presumably to recruit a staff. Authorities arrested her in Massachusetts for fraud and that was the end of her Florida health center. During World War II the U.S. Air Force used the Avon Park facility as a training center for aviation cadets—often referring to it as the "Country Club of the Air."

Around 1947 an Adventist minister from nearby Wauchula visited an Avon Park attorney named Pardee to solicit a contribution to the church's annual Ingathering appeal for humanitarian activities. No doubt the minister mentioned the denomination's medical work. Pardee knew a little about Adventist hospitals because some of his family had been at the Washington Sanitarium in Maryland. He told the minister he would like a similar facility in Avon Park.

Wasting no time, the minister informed church officials in Florida of this interest. They turned the matter over to A.C. Larson, administrator of the Florida Sanitarium in Orlando. Larson invited Marvyn and Marie Baldwin to go to Avon Park to determine the level of interest in the community. While residents knew little about Seventh-day Adventists, they were very much interested in a hospital for Avon Park.

By this time, of course, the Air Force had left, leaving the property in the hands of the War Assets Administration. This meant a not-for-profit organization could buy it for a highly discounted price. The Adventists got it all—hotel, casino and two aircraft hangers—at a 100 percent discount. It would take $400,000 to convert the facility into a hospital, but local businessman Charlie Walker readily agreed to lead a campaign to raise $150,000. The Adventist church promised the balance.

Larson put Baldwin in charge of getting the hospital ready for business. With only three months to get the job done, he scoured the countryside locating equipment and furnishings, much of it from military surplus sources.

Multi-talented Family

Converting the abandoned military center into a hospital fell primarily into the hands of four "pioneer" families from the Florida San. Joining the Baldwins were Forrest and Odessa Boyd, John and Kitty Schmidt, and Harold and Wanda Brown—eight adults and six children in all. They may have been accountants, nurses, chefs, secretaries and administrators by profession, but for three months they were painters, carpenters, scrubbers and window washers.

They prepared their meals in a makeshift kitchen set up in the basement and ate together family style. The women shopped for groceries, and Schmidt, the hospital's first chef, prepared the meals.

"We paid only 50 cents apiece," says Marie Baldwin. "We had wonderful meals—and wonderful times. I can still see some of the children getting sleepy and lying under the dinner table."

Unfortunately, Walker died of a heart attack shortly before the community reached its campaign goal. To honor his leadership and the work he had devoted to the project, the board named the hospital Walker Memorial Sanitarium and Hospital. The "Sanitarium" part of the name was later dropped, but the name "Walker" remained for almost 50 years.

Initially, Adventists planned to offer a sanitarium-type program at Avon Park, and did so for a few years, drawing a small clientele who paid $9 a day for room, meals and one hydrotherapy treatment. Despite efforts to establish a facility modeled after Battle Creek and other early Adventist centers, post-World War II brought dramatic changes to the world of healthcare. Extended stays in a resort-style environment gave way to acute-care general hospitals, thanks in part to advances in medicine and science.

"We went through the transition from non-paperwork and non-insurance to the age of insurance and government regulations," says Mrs. Baldwin.

She and her husband not only spearheaded the hospital project in Avon Park, they also started a church in the old casino. The organizational relationship between the hospital and the church was virtually indistinguishable. In fact, the church also shared the Walker name—Walker Memorial Hospital Church—even though the man for whom the hospital was named was not a Seventh-day Adventist.

The hospital grew over the years to serve the growing community, adding satellite facilities in two nearby communities. A new Lake Placid campus opened in 1982, and the hospital in Wauchula joined the Walker family in 1992. Meanwhile, the aging facility in Avon Park needed replacing. A new 101-bed facility called Florida Hospital Heartland Medical Center in nearby Sebring opened in 1997.

SOURCE

Interviews: Marvyn and Marie Baldwin, 1999.

Chapter 38

Pearl in Paradise

Feather River Hospital
Established 1950

Second Opinion

Knowing of Dr. Edward Sutherland's work in Madison, Tennessee, Dr. Merritt Horning invited him to Paradise to see the site for a proposed sanitarium. Sutherland both surprised and disappointed the doctor because he did not immediately declare it a perfect place for a healthcare facility.

"What's wrong with it?" asked Horning.

"You'll need more land," Sutherland said. "Buy more land than you can ever imagine you'll want."

"How in the world will we ever get the money to buy more land when we haven't paid for what we already have?" Horning responded.

"How did the man in the Bible buy the pearl of great price?" Sutherland asked, reminding Horning of the familiar parable.

"He sold all he had and bought it."

"This is how you will purchase more land," Sutherland said.

In 1946 Horning envisioned an Adventist healthcare center in Paradise similar to the famous Battle Creek Sanitarium. It would offer a strong health-education program, and medical and surgical services delivered with lots of tender loving care. He shared his dream with his colleague Dr. Dean Hoiland and soon they involved others in the project, including Drs. C.C. Landis and Glenn Blackwelder.

These men, along with some community leaders, obtained 35 acres of land from the Paradise Irrigation District for the price of back taxes, $3,500. They later purchased an additional 40 acres for $600. The founders bought the land in their own names, and later deeded it to the corporation that would build Feather River Sanitarium and Hospital. It was a beautiful site overlooking the Feather River Canyon—rural, quiet, and away from traffic, everything Horning thought it should be.

It would take personal sacrifice, commitment from the community and many answered prayers to bring Feather River Hospital into being, but the people in Paradise heeded the good counsel of Sutherland, and eventually obtained a total of 107 acres.

They were ready to begin construction in April 1948 despite the fact that they had not raised all the needed funds. Rather than delay construction, they decided to omit the surgical and obstetrical units. With no collateral against which to borrow, five individuals signed notes guaranteeing principal plus interest. Joining Landis, Horning and Blackwelder were P.V. Harrigan, county agricultural commissioner, and Roy Rankin, retired pharmacist.

Construction progressed slowly as funds came through the generosity of many hardworking people. Rankin opened a pharmacy for the express purpose of benefiting the hospital. Working for only $2.60 an hour, he generated $60,000 for the project. Landis and his wife sold some property for $5,000 and gave the proceeds to the hospital. S.L. Dombrosky from Oakland helped with public relations and fund raising. Many others helped in whatever ways they could.

Ferdinand Stahl, retired missionary from South America, joined the Paradise effort as chaplain. He often called prayer groups together asking the Lord to bless the building program. The following experiences illustrate some of their answered prayers.

The Lord Leads

Horning decided to make a house call one morning in 1949 to visit one of his patients. Seeing the doctor approaching his house, Frank Digital met him at the door.

"Dr. Horning, what in the world are you doing here? Come in. I want to talk to you," he said, seeming somewhat surprised by the doctor's visit.

Digital and his wife said they had just finished praying and had asked God to provide a use for some money they had available for a special project. The doctor's arrival seemed to be an answer to their prayer, and Digital wrote him a check for $2,500.

One woman told Horning, "My husband is a hard-headed old Swede. He will not loan money or give money to anybody for anything."

She said she had prayed, asking God to impress her husband with the needs of the hospital—even suggesting that she would be willing to undergo surgery if that would soften his heart. While she had no indication of needing surgery at that time, within weeks doctors found an *abdominal tumor, and she had to be transported out of town for the surgery. A few weeks later she returned to the doctor's office for a checkup—accompanied by her husband with a $10,000 check. He later doubled his gift.*

འ

Victor and Edith Hoag, patients of Blackwelder, entered his office carrying a round container similar to a large mailing tube. Mr. Hoag ceremoniously began pulling bills from it and placing them on the doctor's desk. As the stacks of bills grew taller and taller, it seemed to Blackwelder that the little green papers would never stop coming. When the last bill had been drawn from the tube, their gift totaled $2,500.

འ

God answered prayers in many more ways than providing financial resources. For instance, a heavy rainstorm hit Paradise at the same time the lumber was delivered from Reno, Nevada. Another prayer meeting was held, and miraculously, the rain seemed to fall everywhere except on the lumber shipment.

The hospital project convinced many people in Paradise that no problem is too big for God. In applying for a license, the doctors learned that they had to have a surgical unit. This seemed like an impossible roadblock—until Horning called the state director of public health. This gentleman, Dr. Wilton Halvarsen, had been one of Horning's teachers in medical school. When he explained the situation, Halvarsen told him not to worry.

Within days, the state had created a new hospital classification to accommodate the Paradise project, and Feather River Sanitarium and Hospital received a license as an acute medical facility with 18 beds.

The hospital opened December 7, 1950. Patients in private rooms paid $16 a day and those in ward beds paid $12. All patients received physical therapy and hydrotherapy as standard services at no additional charge. In the beginning, employees made a personal sacrifice to help ensure the hospital's financial viability. For example, during the first three months, nurses worked for half pay, and local merchants funded the payroll. Zula Ahl, the first superintendent of nurses, received only $250 a month. In addition, the founding physicians gave their professional fees to the hospital.

Feather River was the "first and only" in many respects. For one thing, it was the only hospital in the region that trained nurse assistants. It also offered training for teen volunteers called candy stripers (girls) and handy stripers (boys).

The hospital raised many of the fruits and vegetables served to the patients and employees. Herbert White, grandson of Adventist pioneers James and Ellen White, developed a program designed to "remineralize" the soil and produce highly nutritional foods. This was a big selling point in the sanitarium's early marketing brochures.

Feather River Sanitarium and Hospital was the first public building in Butte County to prohibit smoking, much to the chagrin of patients not allowed to smoke in their rooms, and local businessmen who accused the physicians of imposing their personal beliefs onto the public. The physicians, however, held fast to their position that smoking tobacco was a health hazard and a public pollutant. The "No Smoking" signs remained posted on the walls, and patients smoked in designated areas only. In time, of course, science supported the doctors' position, and public attitudes toward the hospital's policy changed from criticism to appreciation.

Within the first year, it became clear that the hospital needed obstetrical and surgery services. One convincing incident occurred during a winter storm when an expectant mother went into labor. With the roads closed, her husband made an ambulance of his wheelbarrow, and pushed her through the snow all the way to the hospital. The staff had to improvise a delivery room, and having no bassinet, they placed the baby in a dresser drawer. Mother and baby did fine, but no doubt Dad was a bit tired from laboring with that wheelbarrow through the snow!

Outdoors Transport

Lack of a surgical suite meant patients had to be transferred out of town for surgery. Feather River finally added its own surgery unit in 1952. Interestingly, an elevator wasn't installed until 1956, making it necessary to transport surgery patients outdoors. Always accompanied by an anesthesiologist and surgeon, patients were wheeled on gurneys around one end of the building to the surgery area on the first floor. Inclement weather may have occasionally delayed a surgery, but the staff kept patients appropriately protected from rain or snow.

Feather River Hospital was successful from the day it opened because it offered physical therapy, hydrotherapy and health education at a level not then offered by other medical facilities in the area. About 70 percent of patients in the early years came from out of town. One of these was California's 55-year-old assistant treasurer from Sacramento. He had lung cancer and about three months to live.

"I've been to all the specialists in Sacramento and they can't offer me anything. What can you do for me?" he asked.

Horning said they would give him an abundance of tender loving care and make him comfortable with hydrotherapy and whatever medications were indicated.

"I'll take it," the man said.

He moved to the sanitarium, where he enjoyed the extraordinary nursing care and the physical therapy and hydrotherapy treatments. But he wanted no part of the prayers the nurses offered each evening.

"I don't want prayer," he insisted.

The nurses, however, politely persisted and finally one night he gave in.

"Okay, then. If you must, pray!"

That experience was a turning point, and from then on he wanted a nurse to pray with him every night.

Because he was a state official, he received many phone calls and visitors, which began to wear on him. About two weeks before he died, he posted the following message on his door to discourage phone calls and visitors: "I want to spend the last days of my life with my family, and my family is the staff of the Feather River Hospital."

Two events prompted hospital leaders to take steps to ensure the facility's long-term mission as an Adventist healthcare center. Blackwelder died suddenly in 1954, and Landis died in 1958. Although consideration was briefly given to making Feather River a government rehabilitation center or a tax-supported community hospital, the owners decided to entrust it to the Seventh-day Adventist Church to be operated according to the founders' ideals and objectives. Church officials assumed their elected positions on the board of directors in 1960.

SOURCE

Nye, Michelle, "The History of Feather River Hospital," 1999.

Chapter 39

$52,000 for a Pair of Socks

North York Branson Hospital
1957–1997

Help Wanted

The interview was closing, and Anthony Kaytor wanted to know his chances of receiving a grant from the Atkinson Foundation for a new hospital in the Toronto suburb of Willowdale. He had made a written request, and now a representative of the foundation was in his office to discuss a hospital that did not yet exist. So far Kaytor's fund-raising efforts had produced only $16,000, not nearly enough to begin the project.

"How much depends on your report?" he asked the man from Atkinson.

"Everything depends on it," the gentleman replied.

"Oh, please put in a good report," Kaytor pleaded. "We need the grant so much."

As the gentleman prepared to leave, Kaytor wished he had a small gift for him. A pen, key chain or paperweight with the hospital name would have been a nice memento of their visit, but he had nothing like that to give the man. Suddenly he remembered a pair of socks he had bought from a bargain table for about 50 cents. It was all he had, so he gave them to the Atkinson representative, who graciously accepted them.

Likely the man had never before received a pair of socks from an organization requesting a grant. But who is to say they didn't work in Kaytor's favor? A few weeks later the Atkinson Foundation gave him a check for $52,000.

&

A five-year-old weather-beaten sign bearing the words "Future Site of Seventh-day Adventist Hospital" greeted Kaytor when he arrived at the 50-acre farm site about 10 miles from downtown Toronto, Ontario, in 1955. A Canadian, Kaytor had been working for the church in Pennsylvania when he accepted the challenge to build a new hospital in his homeland. Only $30,000 had been set aside for the proposed $2 million project.

"I was asked to be the new hospital administrator, but they really needed a fund-raiser," says Kaytor.

While the church had operated Rest Haven Sanitarium and Hospital in British Columbia since 1921, it had no hospital in the eastern region of the country. The dream of a major Adventist hospital in eastern Canada began to develop in the 1940s, led by Canadian physicians, medical students and nurses. In 1947 a group met with church officials, who suggested they consider the Toronto area. Led by Dr. Erwin Crawford and Dr. Gordon Arnott, who both later served on the hospital's medical staff, the church raised $35,000 and in 1950 bought 50 acres of farmland in North York.

They later sold half of the property for $150,000, which covered the cost of the land and allowed the church to set aside approximately $100,000 for the new hospital. By the time Kaytor arrived, however, all but $30,000 had been spent on consultants, brochures, miscellaneous expenses and architectural drawings, which were rejected by the province of Ontario.

A new sign went up, new drawings were prepared and the name North York Branson Hospital was selected in honor of then president of the General Conference of Seventh-day Adventists, William Branson.

When Kaytor began soliciting funds in the local community, most people scoffed. "We'll believe it when we see it," they said.

On a snowy day in March 1955, selected community and church dignitaries, including President Branson, turned the ceremonial sod and officially broke ground for the new hospital. Kaytor felt a heavy responsibility to waste no time raising the rest of the money for an 80-bed $2 million facility. After several months of soliciting local businesses, residents and church members, he turned to large corporations and charitable foundations.

Absurd Request

Church leaders suggested that Kaytor request $25,000 from the local township, but something told him to ask for $75,000. When he shared this with one of the county representatives, the man said North York Township had never granted more than $5,000 to that kind of project, and a request for any more than that would be considered absurd. Kaytor asked permission to present his appeal in person. Although he was assured he could do this, he was never notified of the meeting. He went to one of the council members to find out why.

"Mr. Kaytor, you didn't need to be there," the council member told him. "Didn't anybody tell you that you have been granted $75,000?"

With large gifts finally coming in, hopes for a new Adventist hospital in Canada began taking shape. Most construction projects of this size encounter some problems, and North York Branson was no exception.

Concrete Evidence

Construction specifications called for a special pre-stress type of cement. Not one piece of structural steel could be put in place until the cement was poured. However, because of labor unrest and strikes at the time, the cement was not available. The problem became a matter of prayer for several days. Then—at just the right time—a boatload of the cement arrived from South Africa. Another company had ordered more than it could use, and having no place to store it, offered it to Branson. Soon trucks of cement arrived at the hospital site and construction proceeded once again.

North York Branson Hospital opened July 7, 1957. In no time, more problems arose for the new facility. For the first month or so, patient census never exceeded seven. There were heavy costs involved in opening the new facility, and the small census did not begin to cover expenses. With payday nearing, Kaytor had to find some money to pay his 50 employees. Banks that had helped in the past turned him down this time. He appealed to local businesses, but found no help there either.

God Never Tires

One day Kaytor returned to his office around 2 p.m., tired, discouraged, hungry and empty-handed. Waiting for him was a man he presumed to be a salesman.

"Mr. Kaytor, I must see you immediately," the man said.

"I haven't even had lunch yet," Kaytor replied, hoping his visitor would excuse himself and leave.

"Well, I haven't had lunch yet either!" the man said.

It was not Kaytor's nature to be impolite, and noting the urgent tone in the man's voice, he invited him into his office.

"Mr. Kaytor, we don't know each other, but I have heard about the hospital, and I have some money for you." The man identified himself as

*vice president of a local Lions Club. "Here is $10,000 for your project.
Will you accept it?"*

*Kaytor did not hesitate for a moment. Once again he recognized God
had met his need—at just the right time."*

Kaytor reported at the end of 1961 that Branson was accredited by the
Canadian Council on Hospital Accreditation—a distinction held by less
than half of hospitals in Canada at that time. Kaytor remained at Branson
until November 1962.

Finding nurses was a problem from the beginning. In fact, Branson
opened in 1957 with only 10 nurses. Working with the denomination's
Oshawa Missionary College (now Kingsway College), the hospital
received government permission to start a school of nursing. The
three-year program offered one year on the college campus and two years
at Branson. More than 260 nurses graduated from the school between
1961 and 1974.

Government changes in 1975 required all nurses to be trained at
universities or colleges of applied arts and technology. This ended the
church-sponsored school of nursing in Canada. Little did Adventists
realize that another change would one day bring their church-sponsored
hospital to a close, too.

"When the hospital was built and opened, it was totally owned and
operated by the church," explains J.W. Bothe, who served as president of
the Adventist church in Canada and chairman of the Branson board
from1962–1973. Business grew and the hospital expanded to meet the
need. It eventually became a 450-bed facility.

Then healthcare in Canada changed. The government took charge of
all hospitals, making sure they remained financially viable, but not highly
profitable. When funds were needed for expansion, the government
provided the money. With an increase of outpatient services, by the
mid-1990s the number of beds had dropped to 209.

Church and hospital officials received the unexpected news in early
1997 that the Ontario Health Services Restructuring Commission was
closing North York Branson and eight other hospitals in the Toronto area.
After 40 years of community service and outreach, Branson's doors
closed and its services were transferred to other area hospitals. The
Branson site was converted to an ambulatory care center.

Adventist healthcare in Canada today consists of seven nursing
homes, one each in Ontario, New Brunswick, British Columbia, Alberta
and Saskatchewan, and two in Manitoba. Among them is the 75-bed Rest

Haven Lodge near Vancouver, British Columbia. After the former Rest Haven Sanitarium and Hospital (later renamed Rest Haven Hospital) closed in 1979, the government invited the church to operate a nursing home. Built with government funding, Rest Haven Lodge opened in 1982.

SOURCES

"Branson Hospital Update," *Canadian Union Messenger*, July 1998.

"Branson Hospital Update," *Canadian Union Messenger*, September 1998.

"Four Decades of Health Ministry End Abruptly in Canada," *Adventist Review*, May 1997.

"Government Commission Announces Hospital Closure," *Canadian Union Messenger*, April 1997.

Nolan, Shelley, "35TH Anniversary of North York Branson Hospital: A Look Back," *Canadian Union Messenger*, June 1992.

Kaytor, A.W., "40 Years of Teamwork and Service," *Canadian Union Messenger*, July/August 1997.

Kaytor, A.W., Report of the Administrator for the Year Ending December 31, 1961, North York Branson Hospital, Willowdale, Ontario, Canada.

Kaytor, A.W., "The North York Branson Hospital," *Review and Herald*, February 25, 1960.

Interview: Anthony Kaytor.

Chapter 40

Golden Days in Sierra Foothills

Sonora Community Hospital
Established 1957

Missing Beds

'Twas the night before grand opening, and the small hospital staff in the central California foothills was busy setting up patient beds. A few days earlier, Dr. Paul Anspach had called the factory to inquire about the missing beds for the new Sonora Community Hospital. He had been assured they were placed on a freight car, but no one seemed to know where they had been sent. Eventually the lost beds were located—on their way to Washington state. They were immediately rerouted to Sonora, arriving just in time for the hospital opening.

Dr. Ben Boice moved to the quiet town of Sonora in central California's Sierra Nevada foothills in 1950. Had he arrived a hundred years earlier, he would have found a bustling gold rush town, populated by fortune-seeking miners and merchants from near and far. While most of the original miners came from Sonora, Mexico, hence the town's name, the lure of gold drew migrants from around the world.

Interestingly, the need for healthcare brought townspeople together for first time as a community. Following an outbreak of scurvy in the winter of 1848–49, they set up a hospital, which operated during at least one rainy season.

Things had settled down considerably by the time Boice moved here to practice medicine. Although fewer than 4,000 people lived in the area, the community had three hospitals: Sonora Hospital, Columbia Way Hospital and Tuolumne General Hospital. Receiving a less-than-friendly welcome in the local medical community, Boice bought Sonora Hospital in 1951. Dr. R. Innis Bromley had built the facility on the main street of town in 1908 at a cost of $1,500. First known as the Bromley Sanitarium, it was later named Sonora Hospital.

Drs. Helen and Paul Anspach joined Boice in 1954, and these three Loma Linda-trained physicians operated the small hospital for three or four years. Other Loma Linda graduates were also attracted to the area, including Dr. Ted Howard, who came in 1956 and remained on the medical staff until he retired in 1992.

"We were just starting our family. We were looking for a place that was out of the way, but not too far out of the way—a place that was beautiful, and above all else, had mountains and trees. Sonora was perfect for us," says Howard.

He remembers the old hospital well. It was a two-story building with a full basement. Doctors' offices occupied the first floor, with kitchen, laboratory and physical therapy in the basement, and the X-ray department and patient rooms on second floor. All rooms had high ceilings, which helped keep them cool in summer. The biggest inconvenience was the lack of an elevator. A large central staircase with two landings provided the only access between floors.

Handle with Care

"We used a gurney when we had to take a patient upstairs. Four people would take hold of it. They would start upstairs, and when they came to the landings, they suspended the gurney over the open stairwell. We never dropped anybody, but I think we were just lucky." —DR. TED HOWARD

Obviously, the historic building was a temporary situation. The Boices and Anspachs decided to build their own hospital. They purchased land on the outskirts of town, and with the aid of federal funding, built a 42-bed hospital in 1957.

Their aim was to build the finest hospital in the area. The one-story facility was the first to have only private and two-bed patient rooms, each equipped with oxygen. It also had tiled surgery suites and delivery rooms, air-conditioning and radiant heat. Patient rooms even had outlets for radio and television. Dr. Helen was the first administrator, a position she held for seven years.

After the hospital was built, more physicians moved into the area. Attracting other personnel proved to be a challenge. Mrs. Boice recalls that effort was made to recruit nurses and other staff by placing advertisements in the *Pacific Union Recorder* and other church publications. While Sonora was in a beautiful and interesting location, single nurses often found it to be a little more out of the way than they preferred, and married nurses needed assurance that their spouses would have jobs, too.

Boice and the Anspachs owned Sonora Community Hospital approximately four years, and then donated it to the Central California

Conference of Seventh-day Adventists. Although they were no longer the owners, they continued to manage it. Boice headed the hospital for the next 18 years, 1964–1981.

Like many other Adventist hospitals, a church and school were established on the same campus. Today's 700-member Seventh-day Adventist Church and 10-grade school are in large part the result of the influence of Sonora Community Hospital.

Over the years the hospital grew with the community. In addition to physical growth, time brought many changes, including a merger with another hospital in town in 1981. Today Sonora Community Hospital is a 143-bed facility with more than 600 employees, serving an area of 60,000 residents in Tuolumne County and parts of Calaveras and Mariposa counties. Construction is underway on a $38 million replacement facility scheduled to open in early 2003.

SOURCES

Benton, Pat Horning, "Sonora Community Hospital continues to offer Christian services to the Central California Sierra foothills," *Pacific Union Recorder*, October 6. 1997.

The City of Sonora website.

Interviews: Eloice Boice, Doris Fletcher Mills (local historian) and Ted Howard.

Chapter 41

Battle Creek Revisited

Battle Creek Adventist Hospital
1957–1993

Johnson and Johnson

When the Battle Creek Sanitarium opened in 1866, Andrew Johnson was president of the United States. One hundred years later another President Johnson signed the guest registry at the sanitarium's centennial celebration—Lyndon Johnson, accompanied by his wife, Lady Bird.

At age 11, Mrs. Johnson had visited the sanitarium with an aunt. She recalled for guests at the centennial celebration her memories of Dr. John Harvey Kellogg riding his bicycle to work. Here, she said, she had learned "the importance of vitamins, sunshine and exercise." As a memento of her visit, the administrator presented her with her original sanitarium admission card.

The Battle Creek Sanitarium under Kellogg's leadership remained on the list of Seventh-day Adventist institutions until 1906. Although Kellogg controlled the facility until he died in 1943, his relationship with the Seventh-day Adventist Church remained controversial. The world-famous San had acquired enormous debt in the late 1920s, and with the depression of the 1930s, it went into receivership. The government bought the main building in 1942, which helped pay off some of the debt.

Board President George MacKay had promised Kellogg that he would keep the facility open, but by 1957 this no longer appeared feasible. Members of the medical staff had either died, or planned to retire. MacKay had little choice but to liquidate the assets.

When Allen Vandeman from the Hinsdale Sanitarium near Chicago heard of MacKay's plans, he drove to Battle Creek to see if something could be done to return the sanitarium to the church. After meeting with MacKay, he notified a group of physicians in Glendale, California, and inquired of their interest in operating it. Among them were Drs. Dunbar Smith and J. Wayne McFarland.

"Wouldn't it be wonderful if we could recover the old Battle Creek Sanitarium, mother of all Adventist medical institutions?" thought Smith.

The doctors flew to Battle Creek to inspect the situation, but before committing to the project, Smith sought counsel from George Nelson, administrator of the Glendale Sanitarium, and officials at the denomination's Lake Union Conference and Michigan Conference. Each visit buoyed his desire to proceed with the acquisition.

It would take $300,000 to get the Battle Creek Sanitarium out of receivership—an amount the doctors were in no position to pay. Two had recently returned from the mission field, one had just completed a residency and another was still in residency. They would need to look elsewhere for financial backing.

"We had been told that we should try to get money from a holding corporation that had been set up to receive funds from the settlement between the church and the sanitarium," reports Smith. These funds were earmarked for medical work in Michigan.

The church agreed to give the physicians $200,000 on the condition that they raise the remaining $100,000. Not knowing where would they get that kind of money, the doctors made it a matter of prayer, relying on the Lord to supply their need, and He did.

Arrangements were made for them to meet with Dr. Charles E. Stewart, Jr., son of Dr. Kellogg's right hand man at Battle Creek.

"I'll loan you $50,000 without interest. Will that help?" Stewart offered.

The doctors assured him it would.

Stewart left the room to let the doctors discuss the matter, and then returned a short time later, offering another $30,000. While this left the doctors lacking only $20,000, it might as well have been a million dollars. They didn't have it. One more time Stewart left the room and returned to their meeting, this time offering to mortgage his office for $20,000. At last they had the money to acquire the Battle Creek San.

Smith and McFarland traveled to Battle Creek to prepare for a court hearing and acquisition of the property. Their colleagues in Glendale were scheduled to join them later. Although all the paperwork appeared to be in order the day before the hearing, the $200,000 had not yet arrived from the holding corporation. Smith called the Lake Union Conference office only to learn that the president was traveling to Washington, D.C., and the treasurer was on vacation. He finally reached the union president by telephone, but little could be done from Washington.

"Time is too short and I have no checks with me," the president said.

"Please do what you can. Everything depends on having the full amount when we meet with the judge tomorrow," begged Smith.

A short time later, the doctor received a call from the president of the Michigan Conference in Lansing. He planned to attend a school board meeting in Battle Creek and would bring the $200,000 check with him that evening. Smith and McFarland waited and waited, but the man never showed up. When time came to go to bed they still did not have the money, and their colleagues were arriving from Los Angeles the next morning. Again Smith and McFarland prayed for God to meet their need.

No sooner had they fallen asleep than the phone rang. It was the doctors from Glendale. They were ready to board a red-eye flight to Michigan and wanted to make sure everything was ready for the hearing.

Without mentioning the $200,000 problem, Smith told them to come. The Lord had faithfully answered his prayers in the past, and he believed the money would be in his hands before the deadline. However, when he met his Glendale friends at the airport the next morning, he still did not have the money.

The group gathered for the hearing with only Smith and McFarland aware of the problem. While they were waiting, Dr. Leland McElmurry, a physician from Lansing, arrived. McElmurry had been invited to join the sanitarium's new board of directors, and the conference office sent him to the hearing—with the check.

The old board members voted in the new ones in 1957. Smith, who would serve as administrator for about a year, sent a telegram to church headquarters in Washington, D.C., announcing that the Battle Creek Sanitarium was back in the hands of Seventh-day Adventists.

The Battle Creek Sanitarium, later named Battle Creek Health Center, operated for several years as a self-supporting organization. A mental health unit and alcohol and drug rehabilitation programs helped to strengthen its financial base. The church took it over in 1974 and operated it until financial difficulties led to its closure in 1993.

SOURCES

Robinson, D.E., *The Story of Our Health Message*, Nashville, Tennessee: Southern Publishing Association. 1965.

Smith, Dunbar W., M.D., *The Travels, Triumphs and Vicissitudes of Dunbar W. Smith, M.D.*, Loma Linda, California: Dunbar W. Smith, M.D., 1994.

Chapter 42

More Than a Hospital for Navajos

Monument Valley Hospital
1961–1996

Jeep Delivery

Hi-chee came to the missionaries' home and announced that his wife was in labor. Without wasting time, Marvin and Gwen Walters climbed into their jeep with Hi-chee and drove over rocks and gullies to reach his hogan. There they found that his wife had been in labor for 24 hours. Despite her situation, there was no convincing Hi-chee to let her go to the hospital in Tuba City. He said he must think about it, and the Walters went home.

The next day Hi-chee was at their door again.

"She is really sick now," he announced convincingly.

Once again, Marvin and Gwen drove to the Hi-chee hogan. This time they succeeded in persuading Hi-chee to let them take his wife to the hospital. They put her in the jeep and began the bumpy 100-mile trip to Tuba City. Not surprisingly, the baby did not wait until they reached the hospital and was delivered in the jeep—literally a bouncing baby boy. The proud parents appropriately named him Hi-jeep. —DR. CARROL S. SMALL

The post office, fire department, water and sewer system, school and ambulance service were all provided through the mission hospital that Seventh-day Adventists operated in Monument Valley, Utah. This was a sharp contrast to what Marvin and Gwen Walters and their three children saw in 1950 when they drove onto the property pulling a 26-foot mobile home. At that time they found only a few hogans and some abandoned movie sets dwarfed by the huge red buttes and sculptured rock formations of the Rock Door Canyon. This would be the future home of Monument Valley Hospital, and here, for 46 years the Walters, and the many missionaries who followed them, would help tens of thousands of Navajos.

The Walters came to Monument Valley at the request of Harry Goulding, a rancher and trading post operator. Having seen too many unnecessary deaths and too much suffering among the Navajos, Goulding offered Adventists land and water to begin a medical work here. At that time the nearest hospital was 100 miles away and most Navajos preferred their own medicine men and superstitions to the white man's medicine.

The Walters' new home was literally something out of the movies because Monument Valley had been the site of a number of Hollywood Western films. The resourceful Walters recycled lumber from the abandoned movie sets to build a three-bedroom house and clinic.

The couple had previously established a school for Indian children in Arizona, and knew their first task at Monument Valley would be to win the Navajos' confidence. Gwen, a registered nurse, began by visiting the hogans, traveling by jeep over the rugged desert roads. Many times the vehicle served as an ambulance to Tuba City.

At first the Navajos were reluctant to exchange their traditional rituals for modern medicine, but in time they began to accept it, usually in combination with their own traditions. As word spread of the nurse's "miracle medicines," the Indians began coming to the clinic, some on foot, some by horseback and some by horse and wagon.

Several mission-minded physicians, other healthcare professionals and numerous students from Loma Linda University gave dedicated service to the people of Monument Valley. Among the first were Dr. Lloyd Mason and his wife who served there 10 years. The Masons arrived in 1958 and within a year the doctor had persuaded church leaders to build a hospital facility. Funds were raised through a special offering and individual gifts, and the Monument Valley Hospital opened in 1961.

Navajo Nicknames

The missionaries soon learned that the Navajo people relate best to people they know. As the Indians got to know the doctors at Monument Valley, they gave them nicknames. Dr. Nicola Ashton, who served 22 years there, longer than any other physician, was affectionately called "Dr. Skinny." Another was nicknamed "Dr. Little Chin," and another was known as "Dr. Quiet."

Even though this mission was physically in the United States, it was culturally a world apart from the places the missionaries called home. It obviously took a special kind of person to work at Monument Valley Hospital. Dr. Daniel Ekkens, who served there from 1968 to 1974, described his feelings of isolation: "...we were located in the midst of a people who spoke another language, who practiced a non-Christian religion which used mind-expanding drugs, lived in dirt-floored homes and had little education. The Navajo also had their own autonomous government. Not to mention that we, too, worked for mission wages on the denominational wage scale."

Time changed things at Monument Valley. Other healthcare services came into the area. Improved transportation made it easier for the Indians to travel to these facilities and they drove their own trucks to the hospitals. Patient census declined. Reimbursement changes negatively affected the hospital's bottom line, with a resulting financial loss of more than $6 million. The hospital closed in 1996. While Adventists had gone to Monument Valley in 1950 because there was no other healthcare available, that was no longer true in the mid-1990s.

SOURCES

Ekkens, Daniel, "American Mission Outpost," *The Alumni Journal*, Loma Linda, California: Alumni Association, School of Medicine of Loma Linda University, Vol. 69, No. 3, May-June 1998.

Ford, Herbert, *Wind High, Sand Deep*, Nashville, Tennessee: Southern Publishing Association, 1965.

Park, Dennis E., and Kara S. Watkins, "Interview: Cyril 61 & Charlotte Hartman and Donald Casebolt 53-B," *The Alumni Journal*, Loma Linda, California: Alumni Association, School of Medicine of Loma Linda University, Vol. 69, No. 3, May-June 1998.

Park, Dennis E., "Of Medicine Men and the White Man's Medicine," *The Alumni Journal*, Loma Linda, California: Alumni Association, School of Medicine of Loma Linda University, Vol. 69, No. 3, May-June 1998.

Small, Carrol S., "Historical Notes on Monument Valley Mission Hospital," *The Alumni Journal*, Loma Linda, California: Alumni Association, School of Medicine of Loma Linda University, Vol. 69, No. 3, May-June 1998.

"The Miracle of Monument Valley," *Signs of the Times*, April 1994. (Written by *Signs* staff and AH/West staff.)

Watkins, Kara S., "Nicola Ashton 64: Captain of the Ship," *The Alumni Journal*, Loma Linda, California: Alumni Association, School of Medicine of Loma Linda University, Vol. 69, No. 3, May-June 1998.

Chapter 43

Homegrown in America's Heartland

Shawnee Mission Medical Center
Established 1962

Unexpected Gift

Months of searching for an affordable site for a new hospital in suburban Kansas City had proven fruitless. Finally, multi-millionaire developer Miller Nichols invited a group of Adventists to look at a prime piece of property that would eventually border Interstate-35. It was a perfect location for a hospital, but the Adventists had no money to buy such a valuable piece of real estate. Nichols, however, had no intention of selling it to them. He donated it—a gift appraised at well over $650,000 in the 1960s.

Nichols developed most of suburban Kansas City. He and others in this northeastern Kansas community, including candy mogul Russell Stover, had high expectations for their hometown and wanted the best for it.

Nichols developed an 18-block shopping plaza—one of the first (if not the first) in the United States—where 400,000 people turn out every Thanksgiving night to welcome the holiday season and witness a spectacular display of Christmas lights.

Shawnee and Mission were two of many small farm towns that were unified by suburban communities that grew up around Kansas City after World War II. For convenience, the U.S. Postal Service designated the area as "Shawnee Mission."

Today it is difficult to imagine this populous corner of Johnson County without a modern healthcare facility, but in the mid-1950s, this was farmland. Certain business and community leaders, however, saw a population boom coming. Among other things, they saw the need for a hospital in the communities that were growing up around Kansas City—an idea strongly opposed by the large downtown hospitals.

Some physicians, however, preferred to practice in the suburbs. Dr. Donald Smith and other members of the Johnson County Medical Society succeeded in persuading the state legislature to approve a bill in

1955, allowing the county townships to proceed with financing and planning of a hospital. Voters—already stretched to build roads, sewers and other infrastructure—flatly rejected a mill levy that would have funded the project.

A year or so later, members of the recently established New Haven Seventh-day Adventist Church in nearby Overland Park were also considering starting some kind of medical missionary project. They had in mind a self-supporting organization modeled somewhat after Madison College and Madison Sanitarium and Hospital in Tennessee. They chartered a not-for-profit corporation and began making plans to build.

Hearing of the Adventists' plans, local community leaders urged them to build a full-service hospital. With no public money available, Paul Jackson, a minister on medical leave at that time, raised funds in the community. In faith, the small group of church members began building a hospital and health center.

After the medical society enthusiastically endorsed plans for the new facility, the community undertook a major fund-raising campaign. Ground was broken early in 1961, and later that same year the health center opened with 100 long-term care beds. Though lacking sufficient income to pay current bills, hospital leaders again moved ahead in faith, and opened a 65-bed acute-care hospital in 1962. In addition, some physicians built a medical office building on the site.

The infant hospital faced almost insurmountable financial difficulties in its early years. Stories are told of board meetings lasting all night, as the directors tried to resolve the problems. Some even mortgaged their homes to raise money for the hospital. Finally Shawnee Mission Medical Center was transferred to the Central Union Conference of Seventh-day Adventists. Russell Shawver from Kettering Memorial Hospital in Ohio was appointed administrator.

Bad News Day

The news could not have come at a worse time for the struggling Shawnee Mission Medical Center. The new administrator was in the middle of moving, and was scheduled to go on vacation before taking over his new position. But the story on the front page of the "Kansas City Star" *on that day in 1972 called for immediate action. A proprietary hospital corporation had announced plans to build a 400-bed facility in the exploding Shawnee Mission suburbs—about five miles from the Shawnee Mission Medical Center. Competition from a large, well-funded, for-profit facility was the last thing this hospital—with fewer than 200 beds—needed.*

Shawver called an architectural firm he had worked with previously, and explained the situation. When he returned from vacation, plans for a new hospital—and a model—were on his desk. The hospital board met to review the plans, and within days, local newspapers published the announcement of Shawnee Mission's plan to expand to 400 beds—complete with photos of the architect's model.

Before either hospital could begin construction, each had to go through the certificate-of-need (CON) process. This was a relatively new—and laborious—requirement, explains Shawver. Both hospitals filed at the same time, and each was eventually approved. In an attempt to stop or stall construction of another hospital, Shawnee Mission filed a suit against the proprietary hospital, challenging the CON decision. In turn the proprietary hospital counter sued Shawnee Mission.

In the meantime, detailed plans were being drawn for the new Shawnee Mission hospital. Shawver wanted to be ready to begin construction as soon as the legal proceedings were completed. Knowing that steel was in short supply at that time and orders could be delayed for several weeks or months, he purchased all the steel needed to build the new hospital and stored it.

"If this falls through, we'll have enough steel to build a ship to sail to South America—and we'll probably have to!" Shawver told his wife.

In the end, the state Supreme Court ruled that neither suit had merit. Both organizations could go ahead with their plans to build. Although the other hospital—called Suburban Hospital, predecessor of Humana and Columbia—had started plans for a new facility, it did not begin building for about two years. Shawnee Mission Medical Center, on the other hand, had bulldozers on the site the next day.

"We were out there with our spades, and we were digging," says Shawver. Shawnee Mission Medical Center opened two years ahead of Humana.

Throughout the CON process and the legal dispute, Shawver worked to develop important support among the medical staff, as well as the community. This proved invaluable when it came to obtaining an endorsement for the municipal bonds to fund the construction project.

The new hospital attracted more physicians and patients even before it was completed. In fact, part of the new construction had to be built above and around a section of the existing structure. This allowed for the care of patients throughout construction. After a new section was completed, patient beds were moved out, and the old structure—enclosed by the new—was demolished.

The new 383-bed Shawnee Mission Medical Center opened in 1977, with then Senator Bob Dole present for the dedication.

"Building the hospital was like pulling a cork," says Shawver. "The medical staff just exploded. Many doctors wanted to relocate to Johnson County."

At one point, demand for beds was so great that the doctors wanted to close the medical staff; however, that did not happen. Eventually the overcrowding was relieved with the opening of Suburban Hospital. Also the newly developing DRGs helped. In addition, new government regulations in the 1980s restricted the length of hospital stays.

In addition to gaining community and medical staff support, Shawver also had challenges with employees, many of whom had worked at the hospital since it opened and had developed great loyalty. They feared the Adventist church would fire everybody and bring in Adventists from other parts of the country. That was not the case.

"In fact, we nearly had to blindfold SDA workers to get them to come to the largely unknown Kansas City area to look at Shawnee Mission Medical Center," says Shawver.

Recent years have brought the hospital continued growth and public recognition as it became known as the "quality hospital" in the Kansas City area. In 1997 *Self* magazine named the Center for Women's Health at Shawnee Mission Medical Center one of the 10 best hospital programs for women's health. The following year the Kansas Award for Excellence Foundation gave its highest honor to Shawnee Mission Medical Center.

Today the original hospital campus of 4.3 acres has grown to 54 acres with a freestanding outpatient surgery facility, health-education building, five medical office buildings, employee child-care center and community fitness course. Primary services include cardiovascular, women's services, surgery and outpatient services.

SOURCES

"There Was a Dream," undated hospital document.

Interviews: Russell Shawver and Bob Woolford.

Chapter 44

Right Place at the Right Time

Hanford Community Medical Center
Established 1963

Interesting Question

The query came in a 1962 letter from D.E. Venden, president of the Central California Conference of Seventh-day Adventists: Is there an opportunity to start an Adventist hospital in Hanford?

"I wrote back immediately, saying 'Yes, I think there is a very distinct possibility,'" recalls Dr. Willard Bridwell, who had been in practice in Hanford since 1950.

Today, when he sees the progress the hospital has made and its plans for the future, he feels a great deal of satisfaction in having had a place in its history.

"If I had not been here when the Central California Conference was looking for a place to establish a hospital, I don't think we would have Hanford Community Hospital today," says Bridwell. "I guess I was just in the right place at the right time."

Bridwell and his wife came to Hanford in 1950 looking for a place with a well-established church school for their daughters, and a community where he could establish a medical practice. Upon graduating from the College of Medical Evangelists in December 1943, Bridwell had completed a family-practice residency, and then moved to the underserved community of Holbrook, Arizona, near a school for Native Americans. In 1950 he was looking for a place to settle permanently.

In Hanford, the nearby Armona Union Academy met the need for their daughters. When an elderly physician in town invited the doctor to take over his practice, Hanford seemed to be an answer to the Bridwells' prayers.

The rural community of Hanford, located in California's San Joaquin Valley, had two hospitals at that time—Hanford Sanitarium (unrelated to the Adventist church), established in 1908, and Sacred Heart, founded by

Portuguese nuns in 1912. The sanitarium was still housed in an outdated structure built in 1913.

In a very short time, Bridwell discovered the local medical community held little regard for graduates of the Adventist school of medicine in Loma Linda. It would take him about four years to gain the confidence of other doctors in town.

Vote of Approval

I remember one physician in particular who seemed to take great pleasure in degrading me at every opportunity he had. I had been in Hanford a couple of years or more, and had gone on vacation when he came to my office for something. It seems that my office nurse complained to him about the way I may have done certain things.

"Well, let me tell you something," he said to her. "Dr. Bridwell can do a whole lot more than that doctor you used to work for."

When I learned this, I knew I'd been accepted. In time, this doctor and I became friends and collaborated on various projects. —DR. WILLARD BRIDWELL

A group of local physicians bought the old sanitarium in 1956, formed a corporation and renamed it Hanford Community Hospital. By this time Bridwell had joined one of the most influential medical groups in the community, and was asked to serve on the board of the newly reorganized hospital.

The aged sanitarium structure—with some of the wiring and plumbing now more than 40 years old—proved to be a big problem. State officials threatened to close the facility if the board did not renovate or replace it. In addition, Sacred Heart built a new facility in 1959, making it the favorite in the community. Competition between the two hospitals persisted for many years, with first one hospital having the edge and then the other gaining the lead.

After receiving Venden's letter, Bridwell arranged a meeting of the hospital board and church leaders. Erwin Remboldt, president of Glendale Sanitarium and Hospital, was asked to look over the Hanford situation and make a recommendation to the Central California Conference leaders.

"Here was a small hospital in a small town, but I thought we could probably make it work if we took it," Remboldt says.

After several months of negotiations, the hospital corporation gave the church everything—the building and equipment, plus all assets, including land that had been purchased for a new hospital. In turn, the

Central California Conference committed to building the new facility. The new hospital opened on March 17, 1963, with ambulances transferring 16 patients from the old sanitarium to the new facility.

As far as physicians were concerned, some of the changes Adventists introduced, such as vegetarian meals and limited Sabbath work, presented little problem.

"They were so glad to have an up-to-date hospital to practice in that they pretty much accepted the changes," says Bridwell. "They were acquainted with our basic principles."

Not all patients, however, welcomed the meatless fare.

"I remember one of my patients insisting that he'd never go to that hospital again because he couldn't get anything to eat," says Bridwell. "Actually, he did go back. In time, of course, vegetarian meals were made optional."

Hanford Community Hospital saw little need to be part of a large corporation of Adventist hospitals when the idea was presented in the early 1970s. At that time it was doing fine as a stand-alone hospital. Bridwell, who admits that he strongly opposed the corporation, remembers it was a difficult transition. However, in his 18 years on the Adventist Health board of directors, he says he saw Hanford and many other hospitals endure problems they probably could not have survived without the strength of the corporate organization.

For one thing, the Hanford hospital was severely affected by a downturn in the local economy. In addition, reimbursement cuts resulting from the Balanced Budget Act of 1997 cut deeply into its bottom line. The hospital also benefited from the corporate relationship in 1998 when Adventist Health purchased the second hospital in town.

Today residents of Kings and Fresno counties are served by two Adventist Health hospitals, 61-bed Hanford Community Hospital, and 49-bed Central Valley General Hospital. Plans are underway to build a 126-bed facility that will bring both organizations under one roof.

SOURCES

Interviews: Willard Bridwell and Erwin Remboldt.

Chapter 45

Hawaiians Wait for Hospital

Castle Medical Center
Established 1963

Kellogg in Honolulu

Adventist missionaries arrived in the Hawaiian Islands in the late 1800s. Sometime in the late 1890s Dr. Preston Kellogg, brother of Dr. John Harvey Kellogg, started a sanitarium in downtown Honolulu, which operated for a short while. Sixty years later and after many changes in the world of healthcare, a local community invited the church to help establish a permanent hospital in Hawaii.

Dr. Robert Chung returned to his home state of Hawaii after graduating from medical school in Loma Linda, California, in 1950. At that time, residents of Windward Oahu had only part-time ambulance service over the old Pali Road. The steep mountain road was prone to rockslides during the island's frequent rains.

Chung was a well-known physician in the community, and part of a small group that launched a campaign in 1959 to establish an Adventist hospital in Windward Oahu. Carolyn Rankin, another community leader, was also a strong proponent of the hospital, and ranch owner Harold Castle donated 10 acres of property for the building site.

The community raised $170,000, and the Seventh-day Adventist Church offered $600,000 towards construction. In addition, both the Governor's Hospital Advisory Council and the 30th Territorial Legislature backed the project.

Even with these commitments, a hospital for Windward Oahu remained at a standstill because the board of health refused to designate the area as a separate hospital zone, thus delaying federal funds for construction.

According to long-time hospital board member Luther Park, the powers that be at that time did not want to create competition for the existing Honolulu hospitals. A series of articles in *The Honolulu Advertiser* chronicled the community's seven-year struggle with the board of health. Unfortunately, the controversy was not settled until two tragic incidents pointed out the critical need for a hospital on Windward Oahu.

First, five men were injured when the roof collapsed at a nearly completed department store in Kailua. The next month, a two-year-old girl choked to death. Doctors in Honolulu said her life might have been saved had there been a hospital operating room close to her home in Kailua. The following month, the state board of health approved the proposed hospital.

The $2 million, 72-bed hospital opened January 16, 1963. Known for a while as Windward Oahu Hospital, it was officially named Castle Memorial Hospital in honor of the man who gave the land on which it was built.

Today Castle Medical Center is a 156-bed award-winning hospital serving all of Oahu. Known for its outstanding community health and wellness programs, it is the primary healthcare facility for Windward Oahu. It was also a 1992 winner of the prestigious Healthcare Forum award for quality.

Strong community support for Castle Medical Center today is evidenced in part by its outstanding philanthropy program. The hospital foundation recently raised $3 million toward a $10 million medical office building.

SOURCES

Judd, Wayne, tape recorded interview with Erwin Remboldt, 1998.

Interview: Luther Park.

Chapter 46

Built on Excellence

Kettering Medical Center
Established 1964

Memories of Hinsdale

When Charles F. Kettering died in 1958, his family decided to build a hospital in his memory on the family estate near Dayton, Ohio. Based on their experience in the 1940s and 1950s with the Hinsdale Sanitarium and Hospital in Illinois, the family wanted the new facility to be an Adventist hospital.

Eugene and Virginia Kettering and their children did not choose the Adventists because of their worldwide medical work or management skills, although these were important, says George Nelson, first president of the medical center. The Ketterings had been impressed by the compassion and quality of patient care they had seen at Hinsdale Sanitarium and Hospital near Chicago. Living only a short distance from the sanitarium, they had personally assisted in the care of patients during a polio epidemic in 1949, and had spearheaded a major building campaign at Hinsdale. They also had met people such as Jessie Tupper.

"It was she, and those with whom she worked, who provided the superior patient care with a skillful yet 'tender touch' that so attracted the Ketterings. They looked up to her as an example of what they thought Adventist nurses should be. To them, she was a modern Florence Nightingale," writes Nelson.

This was what the Ketterings wanted in a hospital to honor Charles F. Kettering. Some months after his death, family members met with representatives of the Adventists' Columbia Union Conference and General Conference. After securing appropriate committee approvals, the church agreed to the proposed hospital. Nelson, who had served 20 years at the Glendale Sanitarium and Hospital in California, accepted the responsibility of heading the Kettering program.

It seemed only natural that the Ketterings would build a hospital to honor the famous engineer, scientist, inventor, philosopher and philanthropist Charles Kettering. Keenly interested in healthcare, he had co-founded the Sloan-Kettering Cancer Institute in New York, a world-leading cancer research and treatment center. However, he was most recognized for his many inventions, including the first successful self-starter for the automobile, a dependable ignition system, four-wheel brakes and the first quick-drying paint, which made it possible to paint cars on an assembly line.

Sometime in the early 1950s, Eugene Kettering and his physician, Dr. Douglas Talbott, had discussed the idea of establishing a research institute and small hospital on the Kettering estate in Ohio. With $5,000 from Kettering, Talbott proceeded with plans for a research center and 50-bed hospital. He employed an architectural firm, and filed an application for Hill-Burton funds.

Sometime later community leaders informed Kettering that a study had shown a need for a 300–400-bed facility in the southern part of the city. For this reason, they were hesitant to support Talbott's effort.

Kettering said he had always intended that the hospital would be built and operated by the Adventist church. A few people in the Dayton community were already aware of the church's medical work. General Motors executives, for example, had sometimes used Adventist hospitals while on overseas assignments. Also, the founder of National Cash Register Company had been a patient of Dr. John Harvey Kellogg at Battle Creek. In fact, he had brought two Battle Creek therapists to Dayton to set up a physical therapy treatment facility in his office building.

Kettering arranged for a group of community leaders to visit the Hinsdale Sanitarium and Hospital. Mardian Blair, then assistant administrator, organized the hospital tour. After seeing the facility, the group returned to Dayton, called a meeting, and within about 20 minutes pledged $1.5 million for a new hospital. Within six months, total gifts amounted to over $1.9 million.

On his first visit to Dayton, in November 1959, Nelson learned that Kettering had opened a million-dollar bank account in his name.

"What a demonstration of confidence!" Nelson thought. There was no organization yet, no written agreement, no building, no staff. The two men had not even met. The next few years, of course, proved Kettering's confidence had been well placed.

Melting Icicles

Harley Rice, associate secretary of the General Conference medical department in Washington, D.C., joined Nelson on a subsequent visit. They planned to meet with physicians of the county medical society who

had been working with the architects on the Talbott project. In prepara-
tion for the meeting, Nelson and Rice rented a typewriter and spent an
afternoon rehearsing answers to questions they anticipated the physicians
would ask. That evening they were met with an icy reception.

"Figuratively, we picked the icicles off the wall as we made our way
around the room," Nelson said.

The chairman wasted no time getting down to business. He
announced that the physicians had prepared some questions for the
visitors. Rice responded with a smile.

"In anticipation of this meeting we have prepared the answers," he
said, placing the typewritten papers on the table. Slowly the ice began to
melt.

One of the doctors had visited Hinsdale Hospital, and related his
conversations with some of the physicians there. They had told him that
they preferred to practice at Hinsdale because of the equipment, cleanli-
ness and quality of patient care. He also assured the group that meat was
available to patients who desired it, but he added, "while the meat was
well done it was usually not done well!"

Nelson and Rice left the meeting believing it had been successful.
The next day, however, brought challenges that took months to resolve.
One of their first tasks was to review the architectural plans.A few days
later, they had found no fewer than 25 major changes that needed to be
made. The plans had no provision for outpatient or emergency services,
pediatrics, air-conditioning or many other features necessary for the major
teaching facility Nelson envisioned the Kettering hospital would be.

Nelson knew he must nurture a philosophy of excellence and
compassion that had attracted the Ketterings to Adventist healthcare in the
first place. It must be apparent as soon as a person walked into the door of
the facility. This meant the original plans for terrazzo flooring in the lobby
with imitation black leather furniture would never do. He insisted that the
interior decoration must "create a warm, welcoming atmosphere with
emphasis on comfort; privacy where indicated; beauty without ostenta-
tion; and, wherever possible, a touch of class."

He also insisted on an auditorium. When the architect said there was
no money in the budget for an auditorium, Nelson paid a visit to the
Ketterings' attorney. He explained he needed the auditorium to help
"create and keep alive forever an atmosphere of gentle, caring, scientifi-
cally-sound Christian service for all who came seeking help..." To do
that, he continued, "...we must have ready access to groups of

employees with whom we [can] discuss effective ways of meeting these ultimate goals."

When this explanation reached Kettering, he said it "is exactly what we want," and Nelson got the auditorium.

The changes Nelson and Rice made to the original plans would significantly delay construction. The earlier application for a $1 million Hill-Burton grant had been approved with the stipulation that construction would begin by July 1, 1960. Now there was no way to make all the changes and meet that deadline. A new application had to be filed, and instead of a million dollars, the revised project received nearly $2.5 million.

Man of His Word

Nelson did not personally meet Kettering until March 1960, at which time he suggested preparing some documents detailing the agreement with church officials. Kettering's response has become a memorable part of the medical center's history:

"What's the matter, George, don't you trust me?" he asked. Nelson said he soon learned "that Eugene Kettering's word needed no extra certification."

Nelson set up an office in downtown Dayton, and hired a small staff—a secretary, plant engineer, director of nursing service and education, and a chief financial officer. In addition to constructing the hospital and recruiting top-quality leaders, he spent a lot of time in the community, keeping abreast of concerns and answering questions, many of which concerned the Sabbath, meatless meals and smoking. Shortly before the hospital opened, the *Dayton Journal Herald* interviewed Nelson, giving him opportunity to also publicly clarify the hospital's position on these matters.

Finding 500 to 600 employees to staff the new hospital was an enormous undertaking. Nelson knew the Ketterings had been impressed with the people at Hinsdale, and that he must bring in a team of professionals who epitomized excellence. Because he had promised not to recruit employees from other Dayton hospitals, he had to move in people from other parts of the country, thus adding to the new hospital's expenses.

Nelson began organizing the medical staff in June 1960, calling together a number of individuals from the county medical society. Knowing they had questions about the Sabbath and Adventist diet, he addressed the matters directly.

"...I explained the Seventh-day Adventist philosophy regarding patient care on the Sabbath; described the Sabbath as a day for healing; and that everything necessary for care, comfort and safety of patients would be done, but that elective surgery would not be scheduled, and all routine work other than patient care would be done on other days...I described Adventist views on diet, indicating that such views were a matter of health, not of church doctrine."

Virginia Kettering played a key role in developing Kettering Medical Center, particularly in such details as the smiling animal faces on the walls in the pediatric unit, and a gift shop featuring many items she personally selected on her travels.

On the day before Kettering Memorial Medical Center officially opened on February 16, 1964, Rice addressed employees and made one of the first presentations in the new auditorium. Following is part of that talk:

What Money Cannot Buy

"This hospital is truly an administrator's dream. You have every-thing that money can buy. You have a stupendous task in the next few weeks of putting in place all the new equipment. You will be completely occupied and preoccupied in testing it and synchronizing it into a smoothly operating service. This equipment is needed to make a hospital; it is necessary. Insofar as financial resources can provide the necessary tools, this hospital is compelled to be a success.

"But do you have an adequate stock of those things that money can't buy? I think of the words of Jesus to Martha when He visited her house: 'Martha, my dear, you are careful about many things. But only a few things are needed, perhaps only one.'

"You have the many. But what are these few things? What is the one? I believe the few things that are needed are attitudes. Boards can vote policies, but attitudes determine whether or not they will work. Money can provide equipment, but attitudes determine its ultimate usefulness.

"People will come here from many different backgrounds and walks of life. The blending process will tax your full measure of adaptability, the tensile strength of your understanding, and the capacity of your charity. Attitudes will make or break the team. No committee can write a job description of these attitudes. No board can vote them. Yet without them the building is but an empty shell.

"'Only a few things are needed, perhaps one.' What is that one? I believe that one thing that can't be bought is purpose—objective. Your objective here? To heal the body and the spirit. Those who come in direct

contact with patients will contribute much. Those who work behind the scenes will be important too.

"Dayton expects much of you. Will you give that indefinable something—purpose, objective, reason for existence—which will produce even more than is expected? It is yours to give. Give to every new worker. Give without stint to every patient.

"You have the things that money can buy. The task now is to provide from the depth of your dedication, the reservoir of your compassion, the storeroom of your understanding, the thing that you alone can give this hospital—the breath of life!" —HARLEY RICE

Education was an essential part of the Kettering project from the very beginning. Dr. Elvin Hedrick had joined the staff in 1963 as director of medical education, and gradually the hospital developed a number of internship and residency programs. In 1964 Anna May Vaughan began setting up a school of nursing, and the Kettering College of Medical Arts opened in 1967.

As his friendship and working relationship with the Ketterings grew, Nelson became more determined to create an institution that would meet their high standards. Along the way there were once-in-a-lifetime opportunities to share his faith, times of crisis and also times of embarrassment.

George Needs Support

One of Nelson's fondest memories of Kettering occurred when Mrs. Nelson had surgery. Returning to his office when she was taken to the operating room, Nelson found Kettering waiting for him. Usually the two men had business to discuss, but this time their discussion centered on faith. After two hours, the surgeon came in with his report of Mrs. Nelson. At that point Kettering put on his coat and left.

Later Nelson's secretary told him that Kettering had come to the office shortly before the scheduled surgery.

"George needs some support," he told her. "I have come to talk with him."

When the hospital started, there were only two small Adventist churches in Dayton and none in Kettering. The influx of Adventists employees to the new hospital created a need for a larger church. The Ketterings would later donate 4.5 acres near the hospital for a new

church, but in the early years, services were held in the auditorium and gymnasium.

Pocket Change Revolt

One of Nelson's most embarrassing experiences involved the denomination's annual Ingathering campaign in 1964. The Kettering church decided to use an amplifying system attached to the roof of a car to broadcast Christmas carols while members conducted door-to-door solicitations. Shortly after these solicitations started Mrs. Kettering was on her way to see the hospital president.

"I met her in the lobby and knew at once that something was wrong," says Nelson.

She explained that she and her husband were receiving phone calls from people in the neighborhood, many of whom had given large gifts to the building fund, and now they were being asked for pocket change. It was embarrassing, and she said the Ketterings would have no part of it.

"If that is the way you plan to continue to raise money.... Count Eugene and Virginia Kettering out, forever!"

Nelson explained the situation to his pastor, and with approval from the Ohio Conference, the canned carols and door-to-door solicitation ceased.

A short time later Nelson received a $50,000 check from the Ketterings with instructions to invest it to earn interest for a project to be determined later. Those funds helped purchase a pipe organ for the new church in 1969. Over the years, the Kettering Adventist Church hosted organ concerts by world-renown musicians and became known as "a place where the best in music appropriate for a church is heard."

Probably no one understood more than Nelson what the Ketterings desired from their relationship with the Adventist church. In his first annual report to the board of trustees, July 11, 1965, he told about a visit to Kettering during a time of crisis. The hospital was out of money. Insurance payments were lagging while the costs of starting up the new hospital grew steadily. Payday was coming and there was no money in the bank. After a sleepless night, Nelson made an appointment to see Kettering.

After explaining the financial crisis, he reminded him of a million dollars in matching funds that he had promised to the hospital over the next three years for specific capital developments. He asked whether Kettering would give the million dollars even if the church came up with only half of its part. Kettering said yes, he would do that.

Next Nelson asked if he would permit the hospital to put $75,000 of his million, along with $75,000 from the church, into operations to help the immediate cash problem. Kettering said that would be all right, too. When Nelson asked if he would make it $100,000. Kettering looked at him for what seemed like eternity, but finally said okay.

By now Nelson was feeling encouraged and thought he'd make another suggestion. Would Kettering put $250,000 of his million dollars in an endowment fund to earn interest that would help secure the hospital's future financial stability? Kettering was rather negative to the idea, but he did not veto it. Thinking he had better stop while he was ahead, Nelson asked when he could have the $100,000. Kettering promptly sent a check in time to meet payroll.

Nelson's comments to that board meeting in 1965 addressed the responsibility of organizations that accept the gifts of generous philanthropists:

Reputation to Uphold

"The Ketterings have given us almost unbelievable sums of money. They have placed their name in our hands. They have some anxious moments about this, and they want to be sure that the program will succeed.... They also want to be sure that the denomination, which has accepted so much at their hand, is genuinely and earnestly committed to the formidable task of causing the institution to take the lead in hospital and related activities and will not let it deteriorate as the years go by into a routine community hospital.

"At the moment, about the only way they have of measuring the depth of our commitment is to involve us financially with them. But they are not primarily interested in our money. They want assurance that their money and their name will be used to its full value in the years to come, and that they will never have to apologize to their friends or their critics for choosing Seventh-day Adventists for this awesome hospital responsibility."—GEORGE NELSON

Today's 486-bed Charles F. Kettering Memorial Hospital serves the greater Dayton area as part of a regional acute-care center also comprised of Grandview Hospital, Southview Hospital, Sycamore Hospital and other related organizations.

SOURCES

Nelson, George, *The Kettering Medical Center: Recollections and Reflections on the Early Years,* 1996.

Schaefer, Richard A., *Legacy: Daring to Care*, Loma Linda, California: Legacy Publishing Association, 1995.

Interview: George Nelson.

Chapter 47

Every Dollar Counts

Memorial Hospital
Established 1971

Biscuit Board Letters

Marie Langdon admitted she'd always wanted to do something for the hospital, but raising $200,000 was considerably more than she had in mind. Undaunted, she converted her biscuit board into a desk, and started writing fund-raising letters, as well as articles for the local "Manchester Enterprise." She eventually wrote 4,000 personal letters—all by hand—on behalf of the new hospital. It took six weeks to raise the first $1,000, and Marie well remembers the first gift—five well-worn dollar bills delivered in a small paper bag by a widow who read one of her newspaper articles.

འ

Modern healthcare came to Clay County, Kentucky, partly to end the famous family feuds that resulted in hundreds of horrible injuries and deaths between 1865 and 1915. One of the bloodiest of these clan wars reportedly occurred in Manchester.

In an effort to help stop the fighting, James Anderson Burns established a Baptist school in nearby Oneida. While traveling the countryside raising funds for the school, he met Dr. C. Adeline McConville, who wished to build a hospital for the mountain women.

Sometime in the late 1920s, the Oneida Mountain Hospital opened. The state operated it as a maternity hospital for about 10 years, staffing it with resident physicians from the University of Kentucky. The charge to deliver a baby was only $1, without regard to the patient's ability to pay. When funding ran out in 1952, the hospital closed. Having heard that Seventh-day Adventists ran hospitals, someone contacted church headquarters in Washington, D.C. Eventually the church agreed to operate the Oneida Mountain Hospital through its Kentucky-Tennessee Conference.

Herb Atherton was administrator for seven years. Robert Pierson, then president of the Kentucky-Tennessee Conference, also invited Caleb

Chu, an Adventist physician originally from China, to practice in Oneida. Chu had worked as a houseboy for Madame Chiang Kai-shek, who paid his way through nursing school at the Shanghai Sanitarium. While there he became a Seventh-day Adventist Christian. He later took medicine and practiced in China before fleeing the country in 1949. Finally he came to the United States to study surgery. Although he planned to return to Asia, a chain of events brought him to eastern Kentucky.

Known as the "Little Chinese Hillbilly," Chu worked from a clinic and traveled by jeep to make house calls. He once said the mountain people often called for him, not because they were sick, but because they had never seen a "Chinaman."

Another Adventist physician, Dr. Ira Wheeler, joined the Oneida Mountain Hospital in 1961 when the charge for an office visit was $3 and a hospital room was only $7 a day. Wheeler worked alone for three months—spending the first few nights at the hospital and sleeping on an examination table because he had no telephone at home in the event of an emergency case.

Herb Davis was appointed administrator in 1963, and over the next 11 years led the hospital through a major relocation and construction project. When he and his wife, Pat, drove up to the Oneida Mountain Hospital for the first time, they were tempted to return to their previous jobs at the Florida Sanitarium and Hospital in Orlando.

"We came to see it, so let's go in," Pat finally said.

The three-story brick structure measuring approximately 50 feet by 55 feet, housed patient beds, a clinic, laundry, physical therapy, lab and X-ray departments, housekeeping, dietary, pharmacy, medical records, business office and operating/delivery room. Three toilets, one on each floor, served the entire building. Patients crowded the narrow hallways waiting to see doctors.

Davis soon learned that hallways filled with patients did not translate into a healthy bottom line. When he arrived on the job, the hospital had $5,000 in operating capital and a payday coming. He learned the doctors admitted few patients because they did not have money to pay their bills. Davis told the doctors to admit patients and let him worry about collecting the bills—a plan that proved successful.

The nursing staff consisted of two registered nurses and three licensed practical nurses. About two months after his arrival the state notified Davis that he must provide 24-hour coverage by registered nurses in order to remain in the Kentucky medical assistance program, which represented about 60 percent of the hospital's income. Davis recruited nurses from other Adventist hospitals as far away as Hinsdale, Illinois, and

Portland, Oregon. Many came from Madison College near Nashville—a source on which he relied for several years.

In time the hospital's bottom line began to improve, thanks to various philanthropic foundations, changes in reimbursement and improved management. With the introduction of Medicare, admissions increased dramatically. At times the 22-bed hospital had 49 patients. While Medicare brought increased census, it also brought a host of regulations and requirements, many of which the old hospital facility could not meet. Davis knew the place could never withstand a fire. Clearly, Clay County needed a new hospital.

After scouting around, Chu, Wheeler and Davis located a suitable property. They selected an architectural firm, had preliminary plans drawn, and the community began an ambitious fund-raising campaign. Things seemed to be on schedule when, without any explanation, the state Department of Health rejected the project site. Davis and the doctors selected a second site, and the state rejected that one, too. After running out of excuses for the persistent hospital administrator, one state official finally told him that money would be available if he were not a Seventh-day Adventist. This was one of many hurdles to jump before Clay County would get a new hospital.

My Word and My Faith

Local farmer Saul Goins agreed to sell part of his property for the project. He was not actually interested in selling his farm, but did so because he wanted a hospital. As far as Davis knows, the state Department of Health never officially inspected this site, which required a bridge for access from the road. The highway department requested proof that Davis had funding for the hospital before it committed to building a bridge. This presented another problem because he had no money.

"All I can offer is my word and my faith in the project," Davis told Jimmy Lucas at the state Highway Department office.

Lucas paused. "Well, Davis, if that's all you've got, that's all you've got," he said.

Davis never knew what Lucas told his superiors at the state office, but within a short time, construction of the bridge had begun.

Time after time, Davis was reminded of the Lord's leading in building Memorial Hospital. One night he could not sleep as he thought about the myriad tasks requiring his attention. He made a mental note that the 10-foot ravine separating the road and the hospital must be filled immediately, and promised to take care of the matter in the morning. When he arrived at work the next day, the ravine was filled.

"I had made no arrangements for the fill, no discussion had taken place. To this day, I have no knowledge of who filled it or paid for it," he says.

Davis sat on a state committee that recommended projects for Appalachian 202 funding for healthcare services in poverty-stricken areas. While Clay County was not eligible for this funding, he saw an opportunity to stretch the boundaries when members of the committee were invited to submit proposals for possible projects.

Experienced Salesman at Work

Davis showed up at a committee meeting with an armload of packets containing preliminary drawings, cost estimate, project description and a full-color brochure. He walked around the table placing a packet before each committee member. Although one man firmly objected, Davis continued around the table.

"Mr. Chairman, I worked as a door-to-door salesman when I was younger, and never once did a man come to my door to buy my product. I always had to take it to him," he said. "This committee has to begin somewhere. Use my proposal as a guinea pig if you wish, but don't throw it out."

"This man is endeavoring to hog up the total project. Give us some time and we can drum up a project also," pleaded another committee member.

Davis could not contain himself. "Mr. Chairman, if this gentleman has sat here with us for these past several months and he still needs time to drum up a project, it is evident that he doesn't have much need."

It was a long process, but in the end, Memorial Hospital received approval for Appalachian 202 funds, which automatically meant approval for Hill-Burton funds. Together, these sources provided 80 percent of the construction costs. The community raised the remaining 20 percent.

Of all the people in the community who helped build Memorial Hospital, one name stands above the rest. Marie Langdon and her husband Roy operated the Kozy Motel in Manchester. On one of Mr. Langdon's doctor visits, he learned that the hospital's request for a federal grant had been turned down for lack of collateral and community action. He volunteered his wife to lead out in a community campaign.

Throughout the campaign, Mrs. Langdon insisted that every dollar counts. She organized box suppers, quilt and craft sales and a variety of contests. There were teen dances, school band concerts, raffles, gifts from the Future Farmers of America and 4-H Club members, and a four-and-one-half-hour closed-circuit telethon originating from the basement of the Manchester Presbyterian Church.

The Langdons kept a goal board on display at the Kozy Motel and were not above asking guests to contribute to the cause. On one occasion, Mrs. Langdon noticed a likeness of Colonel Harland Sanders on a guest's pen when he signed his name. She inquired and learned that indeed it was the famous gentleman of Kentucky Fried Chicken fame. The man assured her he would tell the Colonel about the hospital, and he gave her the pen, which was imprinted with the company's address.

She wrote the Colonel, asking for a donation by July 15, her birthday. Two days before her birthday Colonel Sanders' secretary called to offer his apology for not sending a donation. Marie was disappointed, but not for long. The Colonel himself called on her birthday and promised $1,500—enough to furnish a patient room.

The story of Aunt Sophia's quilt is another illustration of the grass-roots effort that brought the new hospital in Manchester to a reality.

Pieces Come Together

Mrs. Langdon's 83-year-old Aunt Sophia Philpot, a former Clay County resident, wrote her niece a letter. "I love Kentucky, Clay County, and especially Manchester," she said. "I've prayed many times that some day a hospital would be built there...I don't have money to donate...I'm sending you a quilt top...."

When the quilt top arrived, she took it to the Bull Skin Quilters in Oneida to be hand quilted. Then she ran an article in the "Enterprise" *asking for donations. She explained that the name of each donor of five dollars or more would be placed in a sealed coffee can. When donations reached $1,000, a name would be drawn to determine the winner.*

Donations were slightly under goal when Langdon decided to make some personal visits. She first stopped to see Aunt Sophia's sister and brother-in-law, Uncle Jake and Aunt Lucy Sandlin, who were relaxing in the swing on their front porch when she arrived. After listening to her story, Uncle Jake gave her $25.

"We've already given to the hospital, but I'll give on Sophia's quilt," he said.

Langdon still needed $50 when she reached Uncle Holt Finley's place. When she told him about the quilt and drawing, he called his wife.

"Dahlia, get my checkbook and write Marie a check. It is getting late and she wants to go home."

Next morning she took the quilt and the coffee can to Hatcher's Kentucky Food Store where Tommy Hatcher hosted his radio program.

"Folks, here comes Marie Langdon with a quilt under her arm," *he announced when he saw her coming. "Let's see what she has on her mind."*

When she said she wanted to hold a drawing, Hatcher took the can, shook it several times and cut the tape on the lid. Pauline Philpot Massey, the store cashier, pulled the name from the can and announced the winner. It was Uncle Jake.

Langdon and James Nolan from the "Manchester Enterprise" deliv-ered the quilt and took a picture for the newspaper.

It took many gifts, large and small, some given at great personal sacri-fice, and yards and yards of political red tape before the 63-bed Memorial Hospital finally opened in September 1971. The stories of how this hospi-tal came into being illustrate how the Adventist church and a local community worked together to meet the healthcare needs of a medically underserved area. They are stories of faith, dedication, determination and old-fashioned resourcefulness. The people who built Memorial Hospital clearly understand that every dollar counts.

SOURCES

Allen, Jane, "Heritage of Caring: The Story of Memorial Hospi-tal's Beginning," 1996.

Langdon, Marie, *My True Life and Story and Testimony*, North Newton, Kansas: Mennonite Press, Inc., 1983.

Chapter 48

Lessons in Hometown Fund Raising

Hackettstown Community Hospital
Established 1973

Bucket Brigade Slows Traffic

Each weekend for three summers, volunteers—sometimes wearing bandages and hobbling on crutches—collected donations on the street corners along Route 46 in Hackettstown, New Jersey. Money dropped into their plastic buckets would help pay for their new hospital. With many folks traveling to and from the Poconos on the weekends, traffic moved slowly. The Hackettstown Bucket Brigade made congestion even worse.

Sometime later, when the Kresge Foundation made a large contribution to the hospital, one of the officials revealed that he had personally experienced the Hackettstown traffic jams. While the delay annoyed some travelers, others joined the effort. One truck driver, for example, dropped a five-dollar check into a bucket every time he passed through Hackettstown.

At the end of three long years, donations of pocket change and dollar bills dropped into the plastic buckets amounted to over $100,000—more than enough to cover the campaign administrative costs.

As early as 1945, citizens of Hackettstown wanted a hospital. But for many years their interest amounted to nothing more than talk on Main Street. Hope renewed in 1955 when 21 community leaders formed a corporation and personally came up with $22,500 to buy a 15-acre lot to build a hospital. Then another 10 years passed, and still Hackettstown had no hospital. Initially, the trustees hoped to build a modest 25-bed facility, but as time passed, the state raised its minimum requirements—first to 50 beds, then 100. With every change, the price tag on a new hospital increased.

Virtually no progress was made until 1967. A conversation between a local banker, a member of the original board of directors and a pastor/teacher from nearby Garden State Academy led to an invitation for Adventists to build the hospital. Before the end of the year, Milton

Murray, development consultant for the Columbia Union Conference of Seventh-day Adventists, arrived in Hackettstown to raise money.

After visiting local residents and discovering a good level of interest and commitment to the project, Murray visited Dan Allen, wealthy farmer and chairman of the hospital board. Allen had lived in Hackettstown all but six months of his 78 years. Ever since his wife died eight years earlier, he had been committed to building a hospital in Hackettstown. While he promised $50,000 to the campaign, he also secretly designated in his will that most of his estate—valued at over half a million dollars in 1967—would go to the hospital. He shared this with Murray, but insisted it must not become public.

"I live on secrets," Murray told him.

The next day Murray visited another well-to-do board member. Learning that Allen had promised $50,000, this man also agreed to give a substantial gift. Only two days after Murray's visit, the man had a heart attack and had to travel 17 miles to the nearest hospital. Eventually his company gave $80,000 to the hospital.

After receiving several other commitments, Murray figured the community could raise as much as $900,000. When board members asked how he came up with the figure, he said, "You give yourself a margin, say a prayer and make a pronouncement."

"There is only so much research you can do…you have to make some guesses…mine were educated guesses, based on my previous experience," he says.

Murray found that raising money in a small town is quite different from a similar venture in a metropolitan area. For example, trustees usually raise 40 percent of the community portion, but the Hackettstown trustees persuaded Murray to lower their portion to 25 percent. They also convinced him to stretch the composition of the leadership group, and also to include the price of the land in their portion of the obligation.

Still, the Hackettstown business leaders struggled to raise $250,000. When the campaign came to a standstill at $238,000, Murray knew he could not go to local corporations and foundations for large gifts if the community leaders did not come up with at least 25 percent of the campaign total. He insisted that the trustees raise the remaining $12,000 or he could not help their hospital project.

This ultimatum was a difficult one for Murray. He liked Hackettstown, and Hackettstown liked him. In *The Makings of a Philanthropic Fundraiser*, he tells the following story that illustrates his relationship with the community:

Great Little Place

"When I was in town I stayed at a place called the Clarendon Hotel. It was an old building in the middle of a downtown block and typified the inexorable but gentle decline of the hotel in small-town America. The place had seen better days. It must have. The charge was about eight dollars per night. During my time there, the Clarendon slowly began to drift out of business. The number of night workers grew smaller. The restaurant closed. By the end of my sojourn in Hackettstown it was still a hotel, but it was having a tough time. Often I arrived in town late at night after the reception desk closed. I'd come into the hotel by a service door in the back and walk through the kitchen and out to the dark reception desk. I'd feel around in the cabinets until I found a room key, and I'd let myself in. The next morning I'd tell the desk clerk I'd stayed there, and I'd pay for the room. The time came when there wouldn't be a clerk on duty when I left in the morning, so I'd just leave a check in an envelope on the desk. That's the kind of great little place Hackettstown was."

Community leaders begged Murray to stick with them. Allen called the trustees together and although Murray met with them, he had nothing more to say. At the end of the two-hour meeting, they had raised the last $12,000 of their $250,000 commitment.

With this accomplished, Murray made his first proposal to the community's largest corporation, M&M/MARS. When the company representative saw the proposal for $400,000, he "nearly fainted," says Murray. Without even offering a lower figure, he simply told Murray that M&M/MARS "was not in a position to make a contribution."

"It was a dark moment," Murray said when the trustees learned the company's response. "Some of the women cried, and some of the men probably wanted to."

As it turned out, this was not M&M/MARS' final answer. Knowing little about Seventh-day Adventist hospitals, the company sent representatives to California to check out Loma Linda University Medical Center. In the end, M&M/MARS gave $250,000 through a matching program. While it was not the amount of the original request, it was an excellent start to what turned out to be a successful corporate campaign.

There were other hurdles, too. An anticipated million-dollar Hill-Burton grant was cut in half. Adventist churches in New Jersey agreed to give $350,000, and the Columbia Union Conference raised its portion to $850,000. Meanwhile, the longer the campaign extended, the higher construction costs soared. One of the big problems was administrative costs. Not one cent had been budgeted for telephones, postage or paper clips, let alone secretarial help and a mimeograph machine. Someone suggested soliciting funds on the street corners, an idea that horrified Murray. But once again the people of Hackettstown persuaded him to break the rules for them.

When ground was finally broken in August 1970 for Hackettstown's $7.2 million hospital, 80-year-old Allen, now in failing health, could not attend. Murray visited him a few days before the groundbreaking. They thanked each other for their efforts on behalf of the new hospital. Allen thanked the church, and Murray thanked him for his role.

"You led us all to this point. Your leadership was essential to its success," Murray said.

"Well, that may or may not be so," Allen replied in his last words to Murray. "But what I do know is that my having been involved in the hospital has made me a better Christian."

Hackettstown Community Hospital opened in 1973. According to the agreement, the hospital board signed over ownership and operation to the Adventist church.

SOURCES

Knott, Ronald Alan, *The Makings of a Philanthropic Fundraiser*, San Francisco, California: Jossey-Bass Inc., Publishers, 1992.

Schaefer, Richard A., *Legacy: Daring to Care*, Loma Linda, California: Legacy Publishing Association, 1995.

Chapter 49

Serving Cheese and Salmon Country

Tillamook County General Hospital
Established 1973

Family Tradition

Whenever fishing or logging accidents occurred in this coastal area of northwestern Oregon, Jake Douma's grocery truck was called into service as an ambulance. Often his wife, Elmira, a trained nurse's aide, accompanied him to accident scenes to care for patients until they could get to a hospital.

Medical care in Tillamook County, Oregon, has come a long way since the 1930s. Like thousands of hometown people throughout the United States, Jake and Elmira played their part in laying the groundwork for a fine little community hospital.

They moved to Tillamook in 1924, and Elmira worked as a nurse's aide at what was then the Charlton Hospital. In 1929 they moved to nearby Wheeler, where Jake operated a grocery store and Elmira was the community's designated midwife. With Jake's panel truck and Elmira's nursing skills, the couple provided one of the area's first ambulances—a venue of service that developed into a family tradition.

Some years later, their son ran ambulance calls from neighboring Nahalem, and more recently their granddaughter taught rescue and life-saving classes for firefighters and emergency personnel.

Elmira served on a local county hospital board where she was instrumental in developing a nursing scholarship that today bears her name. Little did she realize back then that her own granddaughter would be among the many young people to benefit from that program. Today Velda is a registered nurse and department manager at Tillamook County General Hospital. She and her husband, John, have been instrumental in improving medical and emergency services in area communities. Certainly Jake and Elmira would be proud.

Years ago, when patients in Tillamook needed a hospital, Dr. Robert T. Boals cared for them in his home. He built a three-story wood-frame hospital in 1913, which Dr. Max Charlton later bought and operated until the county purchased it in1942. Tillamook County secured the first Hill-Burton funding for an Oregon hospital, and in 1950 opened a new facility on the present site.

By 1973 this 49-bed hospital faced tremendous financial problems because of declining utilization. County Commissioner Shang Knight recommended that the community ask the Adventist hospital in Portland to consider managing the hospital. Before the end of the year, a three-year agreement had been reached with the Seventh-day Adventist health system through what was then called Northwest Medical Foundation, based at Portland Adventist Hospital.

"Neither party wanted to be committed for the long term, but the arrangement worked, and it was later extended to 20 years and then to 50 years," says Mardian Blair, then president and chief executive officer of Northwest Medical Foundation.

Residents Approve Tax

When the Adventist organizations were invited to manage Tillamook County General Hospital, the facility was in dire need of repair and renovation. The windows leaked and plaster fell from the ceilings. After thoroughly studying the situation, the new management proposed a $2.4 million modernization plan. Even though unemployment in the county was 26 percent at that time, residents voted a tax increase to renovate the facility. The bond issue passed with an 87 percent positive vote.

Tom Werner was appointed administrator and immediately faced the challenge of developing a medical staff. He interviewed more that 85 physicians, hosting many of them in his home. The area, famous for salmon fishing and cheese production, was isolated and had limited medical capabilities. After several months not one physician had agreed to move to Tillamook, and Werner was discouraged.

One day he learned that the Oregon Board of Medical Examiners was hosting a reception for newly licensed physicians. Communities such as Tillamook were invited to send representatives to meet these doctors and try to recruit them to their areas. Because the reception was on a Sabbath afternoon, Werner would not be attending. He telephoned one of the county commissioners to explain the situation and ask if he might be interested in representing the hospital. This prompted a pop quiz about Sabbath observance.

"Is it not right to pull the ox from the ditch on the Sabbath?" the commissioner asked.

Werner agreed that it was, but he didn't believe the upcoming event qualified as an ox in a ditch.

"I know Adventists take care of patients on Sabbath," the commissioner argued. "What's the problem in arranging on Sabbath for someone to take care of them?"

Werner said he probably didn't have a response that the commissioner would accept. "But if I have not recruited some doctors within 30 days, I will listen to any Bible study you want to give me," he said.

Within a half hour of this conversation, Werner received a phone call from a Loma Linda University graduate he had been trying to recruit. The man had decided to move to Tillamook, and was bringing two other physicians with him.

"The county commissioner accused me of having the whole thing rigged," Werner says. "I didn't, but the Lord did. In addition to meeting a pressing need, I learned a never-to-be-forgotten lesson. This is His work, and He will bring success in His own time and in His own way."

Fisherman Reels in Final Catch

From the temporary mobile office where he worked during the renovation of the hospital, Werner watched ambulances and other vehicles coming and going from the emergency department. One day he heard a horn blaring and looked up to see an old pickup truck towing a small boat approaching the hospital. The white-haired driver parked the truck, ran inside and came out with several nurses, who gathered around the sides of the boat. From Werner's vantage, it looked as though they were examining someone, but they were in no hurry to move anybody into the hospital.

Investigating the situation, Werner found that the boat passenger was dead. It seems two old men had gone salmon fishing. One landed the biggest fish he'd ever caught—and then suddenly collapsed. The other man managed to get the boat ashore but could not move his friend. Finally he winched the boat onto the trailer that was hitched to the pickup truck. Bouncing over rough rural roads, he drove to the hospital as fast as he could, but was too late to save the other fisherman. Telling the doctors and nurses what happened, and describing the big catch, the white-haired driver said he had never seen his friend happier.

"It was a great way to go!"

Today's hospital president, Wendell Hesseltine, moved to Tillamook in 1987, and led the hospital through its most recent expansion and renovation. Voters approved a $10 million bond levy in 1996 to expand the Tillamook County General Hospital by approximately 25,000 square feet and renovate approximately 38,000 square feet of existing space. Virtually every department was modified to improve efficiency and service. Local residents, former administrators, physicians and employees celebrated the completion of this major expansion at a 50th anniversary event in September 2000.

SOURCES

Huson, Alisa, "Through the Generations," *Tillamook County General Hospital: Celebrating 50 years*, 2000.

Huson, Alisa, "A Reason to Celebrate," *Tillamook County General Hospital: Celebrating 50 years*, 2000.

Interviews: Monty Knittel and Tom Werner.

Chapter 50

Mission to Appalachia

Jellico Community Hospital
Acquired 1974

Pool Hall Deal

Jellico Community Hospital operated one of the county's ambulance services, which meant the administrator attended meetings of the county squires to make reports, request operating capital and equipment, get budgets approved and that sort of thing. Dan Sanderford needed $20,000 to replace an ambulance that was wrecked in a snowstorm, but the squires were not of a mind to give it to him. They told him to work out something with Jess Longmire, the man in charge of the county ambulance services.

Sanderford knew he'd be lucky to get $10,000 from Longmire, but he phoned his office the next morning. The secretary said her boss was at a pool hall in Jacksboro and would meet him there. It seemed like an unlikely meeting place, but Sanderford was desperate. He gathered copies of his request and budget, and drove to Jacksboro. There he found the pool hall and Longmire.

"I need to show you these requests," Sanderford began. "I need $20,000."

Longmire never took his eyes off his game. "Dan, I'll tell you what I'll do. I'll shoot you a game of pool. If you win you get the $20,000. If I win I'll give you $10,000."

"Jess, I haven't shot pool since I was a kid," Sanderford protested.

"Well, that's the deal. Take it or leave it," Longmire said.

Given no other choice, Sanderford took a cue in his hands and shot a game. To his surprise, he won, and true to his word, Longmire wrote a check for $20,000.

❧

The phone rang late one evening in attorney Don Moses' office above the old National Bank building in the quiet Appalachian town of Jellico, Tennessee, a former coal-mining center on the Tennessee-Kentucky state line. On that night in 1974 Sterling Baird, owner of a local supermarket and a member of the hospital board, was in Moses' office. The two men were discussing the hospital. It was a relatively new structure, built with Hill-Burton and Appalachian Regional Commission (ARC) funds, but it had been closed for over a year due to a number of problems. If it did not reopen, the construction funds had to be repaid, and the board had no money.

"My name is Don Welch," the caller identified himself. "You don't know me, but I'm passing through your community and I've heard about your hospital. I'd like to talk with you if you have the time."

"Where are you, Mr. Welch?" asked Moses, who served as city attorney and member of the hospital board.

"I'm not sure. I'm in a phone booth."

"Can you give me an idea where the phone booth is?"

"It's near the state line," Welch replied.

Moses told him to look over his shoulder. "The light on the second floor of the building behind you is my office. Drive toward that light and when you get here, come up the stairs. I'll be looking for you."

When Welch arrived the three men drove to the hospital.

"I'm not sure what Mr. Welch expected, perhaps a dilapidated facility, but what he found was a new building, neatly kept, but almost ghostly in appearance," Moses says. There were no patients, no doctors or nurses, no telephones ringing. Except for a small section used by the local ambulance service, the building stood empty.

"We went to the cafeteria, turned on the lights and sat down at a table," Moses recalls.

The Jellico hospital board was about to sign an agreement with another organization, but that night Moses, Baird and Welch set up the framework for the agreement that eventually materialized. The Adventist system could loan funds, provide management and recruit needed physicians and staff. The hospital board had access to an ARC grant of about $135,000 if the hospital reopened and met certain requirements.

Later that night, Moses told his wife he had met the man who would reopen the hospital. As it turned out, the other organization withdrew its offer. Moses immediately phoned Welch to find out whether the Adventists were still interested. Welch said yes.

Shortly after the Adventists agreed to reopen the hospital, "the sky kinda fell in," Moses says. The Hill-Burton people decided the Jellico board could not lease the hospital without government approval, and they were leaning heavily toward not granting that approval. ARC, which had provided some of the construction funds and had approved the hospital for a development grant, was also involved.

"This situation caused us to undertake an extensive amount of negotiations with various governmental agencies that held great sway over us," explains Moses. "It involved multiple meetings. J.H. Williamson went with me to the first one in Atlanta." Williamson had headed the original fund-raising effort to open the hospital, and chaired the board when it closed.

Listen To Our Story

The first speakers at the Atlanta meeting spoke negatively regarding Jellico. After listening to about five of these speeches, Moses leaned to Williamson and whispered, "J, we've traveled a long ways and I'm not going home empty-handed. They may throw us out of here, but one of us is going to hit the floor."

"Go at it," Williamson said.

Moses stood up. "Folks, before y'all start telling us your position on this subject, we would like to tell you our side of the story," he said. "You may or may not agree with us, but we want to talk to you. We want you to listen and we want you to listen carefully."

The chair recognized his request, and Moses began to speak. An hour or more later he asked Williamson to take over for him. Then Moses resumed his plea, but he did not appear to be making any progress with his audience.

"I scoured the room, looking into the eyes of the various participants, trying to find some semblance of rapport with anybody. I noticed this woman, Nancy Lane, in the back corner who hadn't said anything. I could see her nodding her head occasionally. I started directing some of my comments to her and invited her to participate in the discussion with me, which she did."

The meeting lasted past lunchtime, but Jellico finally won on a five-to-four vote.

On another occasion, Moses went to Washington, D.C., to face yet another panel of Hill-Burton and ARC officials. Lane, who had become a friend of the hospital by this time, warned Moses not to "let 'em get under your skin." He packed his suitcase and flew to Washington without making hotel reservations.

Permission Granted

As the meeting got underway, one by one each speaker criticized the Jellico hospital as a prime example of everything that was wrong about Hill-Burton and the ARC development program. Finally it was Moses' turn to speak. He drew the panel members' attention to his unpacked bags.

"I'm prepared to stay here if I have to sleep on the floor until I can walk away with your approval," he said. "Jellico has had a bump in the road, and if you deny us an opportunity to succeed now, we will always be a failure. Give us an opportunity. Let us show you that Jellico can be an example of something that's right and good rather than a shining example of what's wrong."

The panel members, tired and wanting to go home, consented to let the hospital reopen, but with a stern admonition to Moses that he had better not fail.

~

Moses immediately called Welch. It was late in the fiscal year, leaving only about 90 days to reopen the hospital and qualify for the grant funds. Moses and Welch arranged a meeting of hospital board and Adventist healthcare leaders to finalize the contract. At this point Welch invited Dan Sanderford, then assistant administrator of Walker Memorial Hospital in Avon Park, Florida, to be part of the health system representation. Sanderford had never heard of Jellico, Tennessee, but was happy to help represent the system in finalizing the contract.

The hospital board members and health system leaders spent most of the day refining the contract. Late in the afternoon Moses took the document to his office to prepare a final draft for a 6 p.m. board meeting to be followed immediately by a town council. Before the evening ended, the contract was signed. Adventists would lease the hospital for 99 years for $1 a year. Each party agreed to give a minimum of one year's notice if they found it necessary to terminate the contract.

"We didn't know what we were getting into, and we didn't want to obligate the health system to something it might not be able to live with," Moses explains.

When a question came up regarding the new administrator, Welch turned and announced, "Dan Sanderford is your new administrator."

"I should have known why I had been invited up there, but it had all happened so quickly that I had really never put it together," Sanderford says.

Welch and the new administrator immediately began plans to open the hospital and recruit medical staff and key personnel. ARC required a minimum of three physicians on staff for the hospital to qualify for the grant. Although few doctors were available in the local community, three finally agreed to help on a limited basis. In addition, two doctors who had recently completed residency programs came from Orlando—Drs. William Oh and Charles Wilkins.

It Just Seemed Right

It was a dark and dreary December night when Wilkens and his family saw the Jellico hospital for the first time in 1973. Actually they were on their way to a job interview in North Carolina, but Welch had convinced them to look at Jellico.

Wilkens was in a surgery residency at Orlando Regional Hospital and under appointment to return to the mission field where he had previously served for more than three years. However, he and his wife had been praying, and with some strong encouragement from Welch, they had begun to feel called to the rural southeastern United States. They did not see much of Jellico on their first visit, but it seemed like the right place for them.

Although the health system had not yet finalized a management contract, Wilkens moved to Jellico and opened a practice on Main Street in August 1974. Many changes have taken place since then. For one thing, two Dr. Wilkenses now serve this Appalachian community and by mid-2003, there may be four. Darryl Wilkens, family practitioner, currently practices with his father. His brothers, Gregg, a general surgeon, and Todd, a vascular surgeon, hope to join their father and brother in 2003.

Welch told Charles Wilkens in 1973 that he could find no greater mission field than Jellico. After nearly 30 years, it appears this family's commitment to one Appalachian community has only begun as the Wilkens doctors continue a legacy of quality healthcare with Christian compassion and a commitment to those in need.

When the doctors and others moved to Jellico, Sanderford temporarily housed them in hospital rooms. It soon became clear that existing housing was not available in the area, and skyrocketing land prices prohibited hospital personnel from building new homes. Sanderford called Moses to meet him in the hospital cafeteria.

Housing Crisis

"I've got a problem here," Sanderford said. "We are sleeping in the hospital and I'll need those beds when we open for patients."

The two men came up with the idea of moving in a dozen mobile homes. Clarence Baker at the C&S Bank loaned the hospital $100,000. Johnny Faulkner brought his bulldozer and graded a hillside that Moses describes as nothing but dirt and mud. Even though water and electricity were not hooked up, employees and their families immediately moved into their new homes, and continued using the hospital bathrooms for the next few months.

Sanderford and his staff wasted no time getting things ready to open the hospital by the August 12 deadline. With only about one month left before opening day, Sanderford noticed that the hospital's license had expired. This called for another emergency cafeteria meeting with Moses.

"We'll just get hold of someone in Nashville and have them redo the licenses," Moses said.

"It's not that simple," Sanderford explained. "They've been expired for more than a year. We have to go through the whole certificate-of-need process."

Moses immediately began phoning people in Nashville and lining up meetings. Fortunately, he had contacts in state government, including a former Jellico resident, who helped facilitate the process. Both Moses and Sanderford say there seemed to be a guiding hand helping them over this and many other hurdles they encountered in reopening the hospital.

"It was like someone said, 'Here are the obstacles in your path. I'll give you the ability to overcome them,'" Moses says.

In the beginning, money was a big issue because it took four months to get approval for Medicare reimbursement. Anticipating this approval, the hospital generated charges and accepted Medicare cards for payment, but it had no cash in the bank to conduct business. The health system had loaned Sanderford $50,000 to help reopen the hospital, but he would have to borrow any amount needed above that. The local C&S Bank had loaned him $100,000 for the trailer park, but that was its limit. Bills mounted as the first payroll date neared.

Finally Sanderford went to see Baker at the C&S Bank, only to be reminded that he had borrowed the limit. Baker suggested he meet with the bank's board of directors. Sanderford knew it would be a challenge for a new, out-of-town administrator to get a $100,000 signature loan for a hospital with a less-than-sterling financial reputation, but he must at least try.

After hearing Sanderford describe the hospital's financial problems, the bank chairman asked what he planned to do if the board didn't loan him $100,000.

"I'll have to go to Knoxville or Atlanta or Orlando. I've got to have some money so I can pay my employees," Sanderford said.

The chairman decided if Sanderford had to borrow from somebody, he might as well borrow from his bank, so he loaned him another $100,000. Then another month passed, and the hospital still had not received Medicare approval. Not knowing where else to turn, Sanderford went back to the C&S Bank to see if Baker had any other ideas.

"I've got a friend down in Caryville at the bottom of the mountain," Baker said. "Would you drive down there if I could get you $25,000?"

"Yes, sir! I will be happy to," Sanderford said. Once again the much-needed funds were made available.

Another Financial Crisis

Although he had heard that Jake McCleary at Union Bank would not loan more than $10,000, the time came when Sanderford needed another loan to make payroll. He stood in line several minutes, anxiously waiting his turn to see McCleary, who was waiting on customers. Finally he approached the counter.

"Mr. McCleary, I need to talk with you in your office," he said.

"Dan, you can say anything you have to say right here," the banker replied.

"I need $25,000," Sanderford said in a low voice.

McCleary rapped his fingernails on the counter several times. "I can do that," he said, handing Sanderford a blank promissory note. "Fill this out."

Sanderford completed the form and signed it. Although he got the $25,000 he needed, he said it looked like a million dollars that day.

By December the Medicare reimbursement due the hospital amounted to over $400,000. Sanderford left town to attend the health system's year-end meetings in Florida. Every day he slipped out of the meetings to telephone the Health, Education and Welfare (HEW) office in Atlanta, and every day the response was the same: No Medicare approval yet. On the last day of the meetings, he made one more call before driving back to Jellico. This time the HEW representative had good news.

"Yes, Mr. Sanderford. I have your check," she said. "Our office will be closed over the holidays, so I'll put it in the mail today."

"Lady, if you don't mind, hold that check. I'll be in Atlanta before you close today," Sanderford said.

He packed his bags, drove to Atlanta and walked into the HEW office only 15 minutes before closing time.

"She handed me a check for over $400,000, and I never looked back," Sanderford recalls.

The Social Security Administration denied Jellico's first Medicare cost report, claiming that it was above and beyond reasonable cost and community standards. The hospital argued that it was a sole provider. Paul Harp, a retired postal worker who dabbled a little in politics and knew many state and county officials came to the hospital's aid on this issue. He contacted Howard Baker, future U.S. senator, who was in state government at the time. Baker sent an aide to meet with hospital representatives.

"We give service to everybody," Harp told him. "We're a mission hospital and we don't turn anybody away. Consequently, we collect only 40 cents on the dollar."

The Jellico representatives wanted the hospital classified as a sole provider, which meant it must be at least 25 miles from another hospital. There was some question about the hospital south of Jellico in LaFollette. Harp explained that the distance depended on whether it was measured across or down the mountain.

"Mr. Harp, is that road ever closed for any reason?" Baker's aide asked.

"Yes, in a big snow storm you can't get across the mountain. You've got to go down and come back up from the bottom of the mountain."

To settle the matter, the men got in a car to measure the miles from LaFollette, down to Caryville and then back up the mountain to the hospital in Jellico. The distance totaled 29 miles. Jellico qualified as a sole provider.

"What does this mean?" Sanderford asked.

"It means you can charge whatever you want and Medicare pays," the aide said.

Harp wrote a letter over Baker's signature and in a few days Sanderford received a check and an apology.

"We were always conservative with our cost reports, so they were not out of line," says Sanderford, but in about six months the hospital was profitable and able to repay all the loans from the banks and health system.

Sometime after the hospital reopened, lightening destroyed the huge air-conditioner that cooled the operating room. The company that delivered the replacement equipment deposited it on the hospital driveway, leaving it for Sanderford to get it onto the roof. Hiring someone with a crane would cost hundreds of dollars, but he knew the city had a crane for putting up transformers, so he called Mayor Francis Payne.

"Francis, I've got an air-conditioner that weighs about five tons sitting here in the driveway and I've got no way to put it on the building. Can you get it up there for me?"

"No, Dan, I can't do that. You're leasing the hospital, and I'd be criticized if I used city resources to help you." He paused for a moment and then raised a question. "Are there any power lines up there around that air-conditioner?"

"Yes, sir," Sanderford said. "The main power supply for the whole hospital comes in right next to it."

"Do you s'pose one of my power lines could get hit."

"Yes, I s'pose it could."

"Well, I'd better come out there and set that air-conditioner," Payne insisted.

A few minutes later a Jellico city truck with crane wheeled into the hospital driveway, and by the end of the day the air-conditioner was on top of the building.

One-stop Weddings

In the mid-1970s, Tennessee did not have a three-day waiting period between getting a blood test and a marriage license. Jellico Community Hospital was the first place south of the Kentucky state line where couples could get their blood tests. They would come from nearby states, and before some holidays such as New Year's Day and Valentine's Day, the hospital lab did nothing but pre-marriage blood tests.

"It was all cash. We didn't take credit cards," says Sanderford.

The couples could go directly from the hospital to the city clerk's office to pick up their marriage licenses. Then they had a choice for the ceremony. They could go to either Dick Creekmore behind the meat counter in his grocery store, or to "Skeez" Howsley at the Union Bank, because both were authorized to perform marriages.

Times and laws have changed, and couples no longer come to Jellico for quick blood tests. But for a time this was a good source of revenue for the struggling hospital.

☙

While overcoming some big obstacles in reopening the hospital in the 1970s, today Jellico Community Hospital provides a broad range of healthcare services and programs for local residents. A $3.8 million expansion in the 1990s included such features as a new emergency center, expanded surgery suites and recovery room, expanded laboratory and diagnostic imaging facilities, modern obstetrics unit and chapel.

SOURCES

Allen, Jane Marie, "The Hospital That Built a Church," *Southern Tidings*, May 1986.

Interviews: Don Moses, Dan Sanderford and Charles Wilkens.

Chapter 51

Dentist Honors His Parents

Huguley Memorial Medical Center
Established 1977

Promised Surprise

Dr. Herbert Taylor Huguley, a Dallas dentist, attended a camp meeting in 1966 where he sat through a long presentation on the church's plans for the Lone Star State. He listened with interest as a speaker shared his dream for a major healthcare facility to serve as a flagship hospital for several small Adventist hospitals in Texas. It would also serve as a clinical site for nursing students attending the church's college in Keene. After the presentation, Huguley approached Ben Leach, then president of the Southwestern Union Conference of Seventh-day Adventists.

"One of these days I'm going to surprise you," he told Leach.

Huguley was considered to be "a man of independent means, very generous with the church and with those he loved." He had served as a lieutenant commander in the U.S. Navy during World War II, and had made some successful investments. He was the kind of person who provided free dental services to needy patients. He never married, and his only sister had died in an auto accident, leaving him the sole heir to a valuable family estate.

About a week after the camp meeting, Huguley prepared a handwritten will, leaving most of his estate to the Seventh-day Adventist Church to build a hospital in memory of his parents. Only 10 months later he died at age 69. At that time the value of the property he willed to the church approached $4 million.

Distant family relatives contested the will. During six long years of legal settlements in which the court finally ruled in favor of the church, Leach said the value of the doctor's property increased "by the hour." Even though Huguley had stipulated that the facility be built in Dallas, the court permitted Adventists to select a site of their own choosing. The doctor's property was sold for double its 1966 value.

Meanwhile, learning of the plan for a hospital in the area, public officials and business leaders in nearby Fort Worth encouraged the church to look in their direction. A hospital would help attract new business.

Paul Pewitt, a philanthropist with oil and ranching interests, gave 25 acres for the project and sold the church an additional 25 acres for $50,000, making a total of 50 acres for the hospital site. Later the Texas Electric Service Company purchased five of the 50 acres for $65,000—$15,000 more than the initial investment.

Unlike the other major hospitals in the area, which were located in the city, Huguley Hospital would be built on a prairie site along Interstate 35W. At least one person in the Fort Worth Chamber of Commerce had some previous experience with Adventist hospitals. Bill Shelton, executive vice president, told Milton Murray, denominational fund-raising consultant, that his mother had been a patient at Hinsdale Hospital near Chicago.

"She loved the hospital, she loved the people there, and when Shelton had visited her, he was highly impressed with the way it was run," Murray reported.

The Chamber of Commerce strongly supported the hospital's campaign to raise more than $3.25 million. An interesting story from this campaign centered on Alcon Laboratories, one of the largest companies in the area, and physically one of the closest to the hospital site. Alcon's involvement was expected to help generate support from other companies.

Fund-raising Challenges

In studying the situation and applying the appropriate fund-raising formulas, Murray estimated that Alcon would give approximately $50,000. Certainly he was not prepared when the company came through with a donation of only $500. He immediately went to William Conner, chairman and a founder of Alcon, and member of the campaign committee. Conner, who was familiar with Adventist hospitals, explained that Alcon did not give to brick-and-mortar projects.

Murray knew this company's participation was imperative to a successful campaign in Fort Worth, and he had to figure out some way for it to be substantially involved. Finally he came up with the idea of asking Alcon to support a health-education program. Conner liked the idea. Murray prepared another proposal, Alcon agreed to it, and the capital campaign was off to a good start.

༒

Huguley has had a close relationship with local businesses throughout its history, beginning with the Fort Worth Leadership Committee, which was organized before the hospital was built. Members included representatives from Alcon, Continental National Bank, Central Bank and Trust, Texas Electric Service, and First National Bank of Fort Worth, in addition to legal firms and area businesses. When it came to fund raising, $3.25 million came from such corporations and foundations as Texas Electric Service Company, The Tandy Corporation, Southwestern Bell Telephone Company, Lone Star Gas Company, Alcon, Mrs. Baird's Bakery, Bell Helicopter, General Dynamics, Amon G. Carter Foundation, and the Maybe, Davidson and Hearst foundations.

Contemporary Structure

Building of the $16 million, 125-bed facility began in 1974. According to the hospital's first president, Bill Wiist, construction went pretty much as planned. One of the biggest problems was dealing with runaway inflation, which made it difficult for builders to get firm prices on supplies. Nevertheless, the new hospital—a contemporary structure of white split block built on a Texas prairie—opened in early 1977, only two months behind schedule and $700,000 under budget.

In keeping with its early agreement with Alcon, Huguley made a major commitment to health education and wellness with the opening of The Health Fitness Center in 1985. Funds to build the 41,000 square-foot facility came from a $3 million community campaign and a $1.5 million grant from the Ella C. McFadden Charitable Trust. To this day, health education and fitness programs remain integral to Huguley Memorial Medical Center's mission.

SOURCES

"Huguley Hospital Celebrates 10th Anniversary," *Southwestern Union Record*, February 27, 1987.

Knott, Ronald Alan, *The Makings of a Philanthropic Fundraiser*, San Francisco, California: Jossey-Bass Publishers, 1992.

Schaffer, Richard A., *Legacy: Daring to Care*, Loma Linda, California: Legacy Publishing Association, 1995.

Whitehead, Mary, "Huguley Hospital—The Beginnings," 1991.

Chapter 52

Miracles of Ukiah

Ukiah Valley Medical Center
Acquired 1979

Small Hospital Faces Big Problem

Owners of Hillside Hospital in Ukiah, California, had no money and were running out of time in 1978 when they called Erwin Remboldt at Adventist Health Services (today's Adventist Health), urging him to take over their organization.

Prior to this, the state had warned that Hillside either be repaired and brought up to code or close. Because it would be too expensive to upgrade the 20-year-old facility, the owners decided to replace it. They even secured an option on a pear orchard that would be a good location for a hospital. Problem was, they had no money.

Although they had applied for a loan guarantee from the Farmers Home Administration (FHA), they could not get necessary backing for the small stand-alone hospital. In fact, at this point Hillside had a zero or negative net worth. Unable to raise the money, and with the certifi-cate-of-need (CON) construction deadline approaching, they turned to the Adventist system.

While the offer was not attractive, after looking over the situation, Adventist Health Services agreed to take over the hospital and build a new one. Thanks to a long working relationship with Ziegler, a leading invest-ment banker for healthcare and other organizations, the health system obtained the endorsement needed to persuade the FHA.

With the aid of individuals at St. Helena Hospital who knew U.S. Representative Donald Clausen, arrangements were made for Frank Dupper, Adventist Health Services chief financial officer at that time, and Dan Ballew, Hillside president, to meet the congressman in Washington, D.C.

"I remember him picking up that phone in his office and talking with someone, and when Dan and I walked out of the FHA, we knew we had the guarantee," says Dupper. "That was the miracle. The hospital had been

working on that transaction for years and nothing was happening. Then it all came together so quickly."

அ

Actually, this northern California agricultural community about 100 miles from San Francisco did not need another hospital. Besides Hillside, there were already two other hospitals in the area, one operated by Mendocino County, and Ukiah General Hospital, owned by Hospital Corporation of America (HCA).

When dentist Donal Anderson moved to Ukiah in the early 1950s, only eight or 10 physicians practiced in the community. Perhaps half were Seventh-day Adventists. He describes the hospital as "quite an antique." For one thing, scrubs were not used in the operating rooms. Anderson, longtime board member of Ukiah Valley Medical Center, recalls having to wear a facemask to extract teeth, but no other special surgical attire was required. One time he saw another physician performing a tonsillectomy in his undershirt—of course, also wearing the mandatory facemask.

Tensions began to mount as the Adventist physicians found their surgery schedules frequently changed without notice. Then Dr. Robert Barr built Hillside Hospital in 1956.

"It was not an Adventist hospital, but because it was supported by the Adventist doctors in town, it was called an Adventist hospital," explains Anderson.

When Barr went bankrupt, the physicians and others came to the hospital's rescue in 1960, and operated it as a not-for-profit hospital for several years. In the meantime, HCA purchased Ukiah General and built a new facility. When it appeared in the late 1970s that Hillside would not get financial backing to rebuild, it seemed only a matter of time until the old facility would close, leaving Ukiah General as the sole non-government hospital in town.

Hillside's future took another downturn when the administrator resigned. The board then invited Dan Ballew from Portland Adventist Hospital in Oregon to be administrator. Ballew knew that a relationship with the Adventist system could help the struggling Ukiah hospital.

Proponents of Ukiah General did their best to keep Hillside from rebuilding. A negative campaign was launched—with heated town meetings and negative newspaper ads—attempting to keep the Adventist system out of the community. Among other things claims were made that Adventists would provide no medical care between sunset Friday and sunset Saturday, that they would attempt to proselytize, and would not serve meat in the hospital.

"Somehow we got through all that and rallied enough support from the community and our board that we were able to move ahead," says Remboldt.

During the 17-month construction period, Ballew and chief financial officer Jim Brewster managed to reverse Hillside's losses. Within two years of opening the new hospital in 1980, it also had a positive balance sheet.

More changes lay ahead for the hospitals in this community. Ukiah General was one of several HCA hospitals spun off to form a new company called HealthTrust. Also, the county hospital eventually discontinued its acute-care business. As time went on, it became increasingly clear that Ukiah needed only one hospital. The question was, which one? Unknown to the community, HealthTrust and the Adventist system had begun negotiating a resolution to the problem. This ultimately led to the Adventists purchasing Ukiah General in 1988.

"The announcement was a stunning surprise to the community," says Don Ammon, today's president of Adventist Health, who represented the Adventist system in the transaction. "Negotiations had gone on for about five months and nobody leaked it."

Not surprisingly, some people were very upset, and the matter wasn't resolved until after a lengthy Federal Trade Commission challenge. In the end, the Adventist hospital won and the combined facilities were renamed Ukiah Valley Medical Center.

While the transition has taken time, Ammon says Ukiah Valley Medical Center has a good medical staff today. After providing services at both facilities for more than 10 years, all hospital operations were recently consolidated on the site built in 1980. The county purchased the second plant for its public health services. With nearly 100 patient beds, Ukiah Valley Medical Center serves an area with over 60,000 residents.

SOURCES

"Ukiah Adventist Hospital: Brief Outline of History," 1985.

"Ukiah General Hospital," undated document.

"Ukiah Valley Medical Center History," 2000.

"Ukiah Valley Medical Center: Our History, Culture and Expectations," undated.

Interviews: Don Ammon, Donal Anderson, Frank Dupper, Richard Guthrie, Don Jernigan and Erwin Remboldt.

Chapter 53

Shuffleboard Courts and Fitness Trails

East Pasco Medical Center
Established 1985

Hilltop Site Selected

When time came to buy property to build a replacement hospital, Don Welch, then president of Adventist Health System/Sunbelt, and Bob Scott, executive vice president, invited Bob Wade to go with them to look at potential sites around Zephyrhills. As their small plane flew over a large hill of several acres overlooking Highway 301, Welch declared it was the right spot for the hospital. He had no interest in considering any other properties in the area.

"Snowbirds" have been flocking to Zephyrhills, Florida, for decades. Mobile home parks, shuffleboard and visits to local orange groves offered relief from frigid winter temperatures for thousands of retirees from "Up North."

The 52-bed Jackson Memorial Hospital in a residential section of Dade City had served the county for many years, but serious cases had to go out-of-town. When local osteopathic physicians W.E. Stanfield and Marcelino Oliva succeeded in their lawsuit to gain admittance to the hospital medical staff, some local physicians did not take lightly to the ruling. They left Jackson Memorial and built a facility in Dade City, which was known for many years as "Doctors' Hospital."

Because Jackson Memorial was the county hospital, Doctors' Hospital physicians avoided caring for indigent patients, many of whom were migrant workers in the citrus business. They were young families, which accounted for a high number of uninsured obstetrics cases. The result was a steadily declining bottom line that eventually forced the county to put the hospital on the market in 1981. One of the physicians called Bob Scott in Orlando.

"Why haven't you folks submitted a proposal?" he asked.

"We didn't know the hospital was for sale," Scott told him.

Proposals had to be in by the end of the week, which was not an overwhelming obstacle because Scott had prepared dozens of similar proposals. Before agreeing to make a proposal, he met with the medical staff, which agreed to support him 100 percent.

In looking at the situation, Welch, Scott and others at the Adventist corporate office recognized a potential population boom in the area. With its close proximity to Tampa and the growing retiree population, it appeared to have potential.

Of about a dozen proposals submitted, the hospital board took only two to the county commissioners for final selection—Humana, which operated Doctors' Hospital, and Adventist Health System. In the meantime, Scott and the local Adventist minister, Larry Groger, began visiting some of the movers and shakers in the community.

"This pastor was incredible. He knew everybody in the courthouse. He was a member of Kiwanis, and he was a chaplain for the sheriff's department," says Scott. "There was no place we went that he didn't know the people."

Prior to the meeting of the county commissioners, a boy was injured on a school playground and taken to the Doctors' Hospital emergency department. Scott recalls that he had broken an arm or leg—but his family had no insurance. After six or seven hours of waiting, he was transferred to another hospital for treatment. When the story hit the newspaper, people were upset. Someone asked Scott what he would have done and he said, "I'd take care of the kid first, and worry about the money later."

Finally time came for Humana and the Adventists to present their proposals to the commissioners. Scott knew Humana had the advantage because it already operated one hospital in the area. Also, Scott was scheduled to make his presentation first, giving Humana opportunity to respond to his comments. However, after each had presented his material, the chairman asked them for final statements—with the speakers in reverse order.

The Humana representative said the community needed only one hospital. Scott knew that was true, but figured he'd give it his best shot.

Adventists Win Vote

"I couldn't help but listen to what this gentleman told you," he began. "And quite frankly, the man is right. I've discussed that very matter with the doctors. They agree. They just don't want it to be Humana. I wonder if you'd vote for us if they would agree to sell."

Someone in the room shouted "Yes!" and Scott sat down. The vote was overwhelmingly in favor of the Adventist system.

Adventists leased the old facility with the understanding they would build a replacement hospital in nearby Zephyrhills, provided they could obtain approval for additional beds. In the meantime, the health system would refurbish the old hospital and reopen services such as obstetrics and the emergency department, as well as continue providing indigent care.

Bob Wade transferred from Florida Hospital to oversee the transition from Dade City to Zephyrhills. He arrived on the job in May 1981 to find three patients in the hospital and a medical staff of seven.

Paint Brushes for All

As part of the purchase deal, the health system had promised the employees could keep their jobs. With only three patients in the hospital, what was Wade to do with all the nurses, therapists, housekeepers, engineers and other employees? He put brushes in their hands and put them to work painting the old building.

A coat of paint and new carpeting gave the old place a fresh look, but Wade needed physicians and patients. The corporate office assisted in recruiting physicians, and in time the 53-bed hospital was operating at full capacity. It received its first accreditation in November 1982.

Indeed, things improved. However, the indigent business continued to erode the bottom line, leading critics to question the wisdom of getting involved in what was sometimes referred to as "Welch and Scott's Folly."

By the time the Adventist system submitted its certificate-of-need application, Humana had already filed theirs. Also the state had changed the rules. Instead of applications being considered monthly, it was done only twice a year. Since the two hospitals were competing for the same beds, the Adventists needed to submit an application in time to be considered with Humana's. With three days remaining before the deadline, Scott flew to St. Louis, Missouri, met with the contractor, and spent the next day designing the first phase of the building. The following day the contractor had a price to submit with the certificate of need.

The Humana representatives never dreamed the Adventist system could meet the deadline. Meanwhile, one of Scott's acquaintances with the state of Florida telephoned him.

"Bob I've got a problem. Technically you qualify for those beds, but I'm getting a lot of heat from the governor. Is there any way you guys can compromise?"

Scott met with a Humana representative and offered to give up 10 beds if Doctors' Hospital would do the same, but he wouldn't agree to it. The matter ended up in the hands of attorneys and instead of 100 beds, Adventists got only 85.

Ground was broken in October 1982, with then Florida Governor Bob Graham as the keynote speaker. In a campaign called Heartbeat 83, the community raised $750,000 for a cardiac-care unit and emergency department—even though some said it would be impossible to raise that kind of money in a retirement community where most residents migrated north every summer.

Construction proceeded on the $17 million medical center—financed entirely by the health system. Wade says things went fairly smoothly except for a huge hole in the ground, which had to be filled with thousands of yards of concrete.

Part of the indigent care problem resolved itself after a devastating freeze that wiped out much of the area's citrus industry, reducing the need for migrant workers. However, a sizable indigent population still remained, and young families and retirees continued moving to the area.

The new East Pasco Medical Center opened in February 1985 with nearly 50 physicians on staff. Every hospital bed was filled within 72 hours. With the transition from the old to the new completed, Wade returned to Florida Hospital and Roy Orr became president of East Pasco Medical Center.

Even though it was a brand new facility the medical center carried the stigma of the old county hospital. Orr set out to change that. Among other things, he initiated three programs that continue today—an Easter sunrise service, a "Lifesaver Picnic" for emergency medical services, firefighters and police (which now also includes hospital employees), and a Christmas-tree-decorating program on the hospital lawn. Nicknamed "A Stately Affair" by future hospital president Bob Dodd, members of the community decorate the trees in themes representing their home states or provinces.

Shelter in a Storm

When Hurricane Elena threatened the area's many mobile home residents in 1985, Orr opened the hospital as a community shelter. Hundreds of people found safety, warm food and a place to sleep at the new hospital, marking a turning point in the public's perception. The Zephyrhills hospital was new, well equipped and friendly, too.

Local residents soon began embracing East Pasco Medical Center as their hospital.

❧

Bob Dodd was appointed president in 1986, facing a medical staff and group of employees who did not know what to expect of the new administration. By this time competition from the other hospital had grown hostile.

"As I thought about a guiding philosophy, I thought of Christ and the Golden Rule: 'Do unto others as you would have them do unto you,'" Dodd recalls.

Wade had overseen closure of the old county hospital and construction of the new facility. Orr had built strong bridges to the community. Dodd needed to develop the mission and Christian culture.

During the next 11 years the hospital established many new programs and crossed new bridges. The facility grew from 85,000 to 240,000 square feet and from 85 to 120 patient beds. The staff grew from less than 50 physicians to about 150.

The matter of indigent care was somewhat alleviated by a federally funded clinic in Dade City. Unfortunately, the clinic had high physician turnover, quality of care declined and funding was soon depleted. East Pasco Medical Center took most of the indigent maternity cases, but sorely needed a financially viable plan for caring for these patients.

Claire Warner, vice president for patient care, came up with the idea of a midwifery clinic, which was successful from the beginning. Within a short time the staff of eight midwives reported the lowest infant mortality rate in Florida. It later joined operations with another clinic in the area.

Accommodating Patient Overflow

While the state limited the number of licensed beds for each hospital, it did not limit the number of patients a hospital could care for at any given time. Every winter, when the northern snowbirds returned to Florida, East Pasco Medical Center faced a severe bed shortage. To help accommodate the overflow, Dodd and Warner came up with the idea of an observation unit for patients to stay up to 24 hours prior to admission. These beds did not count in the hospital's total licensed beds. Also, the addition of an 11-bed skilled nursing unit based in the hospital further helped alleviate the problem.

❧

East Pasco Medical Center began various efforts to promote wellness and preventive medicine. One of the most successful was a fitness trail on the hospital's spacious front lawn. Mothers pushing baby carriages, cardiac patients stepping out for their daily exercise, as well as fitness buffs seeking a good aerobic workout are regularly seen walking or jogging around the trail. The park-like surroundings are well lighted, providing a pleasant and safe place to exercise day or night.

When time came to expand the outpatient surgery facilities, Dodd wanted the new construction linked to the existing hospital. The architect came up with a design that created a spacious main entrance between the new and old structures. The spiritual life committee suggested using that space to illustrate the hospital's mission. The result is a two-story mural, a sculpture of Christ holding a child, and a three-story column bearing bronze sculptures of a series of hands that evolve into a dove.

Dodd explains that the hands and dove depict "many hands working together under the influence of the Holy Spirit."

Silent Witness

A patient watched silently from the walkway outside his room in the progressive-care unit while artist Andy Davenport painted the colorful mural in the new hospital lobby. Day after day he followed the artist's brush revealing inspirational images of life and health in the Florida sunshine—images that would help form visitors' first impressions when they entered the building. Later the patient said that watching the painting come into being had had a significant effect on his recovery.

East Pasco Medical Center has come a long way since the day the health system purchased the old county hospital in 1981. It continues to develop into a regional medical center, expecting to reach a total of 250 to 300 beds by 2005.

SOURCES

"East Pasco Medical Center," 1999.

"The EPMC Hands," undated.

Interviews: Bob Dodd, Bob Scott, Bob Wade and Claire Warner.

Chapter 54

Fountain Pen Legacy

Florida Hospital Waterman
Acquired 1992

Fashionable Hotel

During the Florida land boom in the 1920s, Frank Waterman, president of Waterman Fountain Pen Company, built the Fountain Inn in downtown Eustis, about 30 miles north of Orlando. The fashionable hotel drew many guests, especially residents of the northern states during the winter months. Unfortunately, like many other enterprises, the inn suffered financially when the land boom ended after the 1929 stock market crash. In 1938 Waterman offered part of his hotel to a group of local physicians for a hospital.

Healthcare had been a concern for Lake County residents for several years. According to a 1926 newspaper report, the county had no provision to care for its sick or injured. Hospitals in adjoining counties were full and unable to care for cases from Lake County. Then in 1933 Dr. W.L. Ashton opened the 18-bed Lake County Medical Center, sharing a hotel in nearby Umatilla with the Florida Elks' home for handicapped children.

With Waterman's offer, Ashton moved the hospital to Eustis, this time sharing quarters with a bank, drug store, grocery store, barbershop, dentist's office and for a time, a bar. One floor continued to serve hotel guests, and for a while hospital employees lived on the third floor.

A series of expansions over the years changed the appearance of the downtown Eustis facility as it grew into a modern hospital accommodating 182 patient beds and new services and technology. Trustees changed the name, too, first to Waterman Memorial Hospital, and then Waterman Medical Center. More changes would be necessary for the hospital to remain viable and continue to meet the healthcare needs of Lake County.

With the changing healthcare environment of the early 1990s, hospital leaders recognized the need to join a larger organization. They looked to Florida Hospital, a tertiary-level Adventist facility that had served neighboring Orange and Seminole counties since 1908. Adventist Health

System assumed ownership of Waterman Medical Center in 1992, and subsequently renamed it Florida Hospital Waterman. Construction began in 2000 on a facility to replace the aging downtown plant, thus ensuring the Waterman legacy continues to provide healthcare services to Lake County residents for many years to come.

SOURCE

Johnson, Miriam, "Lake County's First Hospital," reprinted from Lake County Historical Society newsletter, January 1, 1989, in a supplement to *Triangle Shopping Guide*, August 6, 1997.

Part 4

Appendix

Appendix A

Why SDA Hospitals?

By
*George Nelson**

"To introduce this presentation I wish to borrow from my friend, the late, great Harley Rice; poet, philosopher, world traveler, author. In the field of leadership, especially health care administration, he was a giant.

"The medical ministry of the church," he once wrote, "is made up of ideas, people, and things. The things—bricks and mortar, equipment, machinery—are probably the least important of the three, though things are indispensable. An idea or a conviction without people is but an academic profundity. It requires people to give ideas and convictions the breath of life. The medical ministry of the church finds its fulfillment only through the lives of people. The joy of contributing to the success of the church in its great ministry of salvation; the quiet satisfaction at the end of the day of having done good and faithful work to lessen the sorrows of mankind; the happiness of feeling that one is involved in a joint endeavor with the Great Physician and in being lost in something bigger than oneself is beyond price....

"By its very nature, the contact is made when people are sick and often in pain. These are times when they are prone to be thinking about the serious values of life. In times of acute illness, when one is laid low, (s)he may realize that life is brief at best. Such an awareness causes one to think about the great hereafter and to measure life by its values which are truer than money or possessions. Thus, the medical ministry of the church in its widest application—and that includes every person who helps to make up the Adventist medical ministry—tends to reach people in their more serious moments, when the door of the heart is more likely to be ajar. At the bedside in the quiet of evening one can say, 'How long we live is not all that counts. How well we live is also important. God promises a life beyond the brevity of our years here....'"

"Adventist medical ministry is unique only when it combines science with compassion, competence with love, and skill with understanding and sympathy. When these are combined, the world takes notice....

"Christ's love and sympathy, His understanding, compassion and healing spoke for itself, and multitudes heard and followed. In the world today there is still that desperate need for love, for sympathy, for understanding, for compassion. Hearts ache and tears flow for lack of these elements as much as for causes born of physical pain. These needs are as old as history and date back to the first funeral service on earth and to the first crop of thistles that ever cast their seed on tear-spattered sod."

"In denominational publications many references are made to our medical institutions and their purposes. I think, however, that the substance of all the counsels is well stated in a single sentence: 'Our medical institutions are established to relieve the sick and the afflicted, to awaken a sprit of inquiry, to disseminate light, and to advance reform.'

"What a marvelous statement! In our medical institutions we should put forth strong endeavor to carry out these principles. In order to do this by way of an organization, it is necessary that all those who share in the program understand its purpose, for the spirit of an institution is found not only in its physical facilities but in the attitudes, the personalities, the will and the dedication of its people.

"The first purpose is very clear—to relieve the sick and the afflicted. The second—to awaken a spirit of inquiry, puzzled me a little at first, but the more I have thought about it over the years, the more value and wisdom I see in it. It is a stimulus to create an atmosphere that is so appealing, so striking, so different, that people will not at first understand it, but will be impressed by it. This purpose is achieved, not so much by what is said as by what is done. Though it is important to know what to say, it is very important to know what not to say. What a richness there might be to our influence if all could be engulfed in an atmosphere of Christian love and dignity, and in that pervading atmosphere work with quiet, cheerful, dignified efficiency. In such circumstances our words, our actions, our work, our attitudes and the atmosphere surrounding us may cause others to ask: 'What causes the influence I am experiencing here?' 'What is different about this place?'; 'Why is Saturday a quiet day here?'; 'Why do you recommend that I modify my diet?' Perhaps some might even be inclined to ask, 'What shall I do to be saved?' Maybe we need to ask ourselves that last question. When John the Baptist was preaching in the desert near Jerusalem, some of the people who heard him asked, 'What shall we do to be saved?' John answered, 'He that hath two coats, let him impart to him that hath none; and he that hath meat, let him do likewise.' In other words, be generous.

"*Others who asked that same question were the publicans, the tax gatherers who had bought the right to exact as much as possible from the people in that district, retaining any surplus they might collect as their own property. John's response to these men was clear, honest, forthright. 'Exact no more than that which is appointed you.' In other words, be honest and fair.*

"*Then came the soldiers—we are all soldiers of the cross—and maybe John's answer to their question about what they should do to be saved has a special application to us. His reply to them was, 'Do violence to no man, neither accuse any falsely; and be content with your wages.' This is all! It was just as simple as that.*

"*In modern English, be kind, stop criticizing, and be content. Even more tersely said, 'Stop fussing and complaining about others, and be satisfied.' If we do just that, it is likely that more and more will ask us, 'What shall I do to be saved?'*

"*Thirdly, the hospital and its people should disseminate light. When a spirit of inquiry has been awakened in the minds of those who see or receive the ministry of healing, it should be possible to answer their questions in a way that will properly cause light to shine where darkness existed.*

"*An area in which the hospital must disseminate light is in teaching the principles of healthful living. This is done by individual example and advice, by classes of instruction for personnel, and by public programs conducted by trained health workers from many sections of the hospital complex...*

"*The fourth great purpose is to advance reform. What is reform? It is to change into a new form, to amend, to improve, to change. It is the opposite of stagnation. In the sense in which it is used here, it means to retain what is good from the past, and accept what is proved to be good from the new. This is not counsel that applies to a given time and situation. It is living instruction. It means the same today that it meant 75 years ago. It means ADVANCE! Move forward! Don't stand still! Advance change!*

"*Now, just a few words about the effect of the medical institutions upon the church at large, in ways I have not so far mentioned directly. I shall use the Kettering Medical Center for illustration.*

"*When I arrived in the Dayton-Kettering community, there were two Adventist churches...with about 150 members. The funds flowing to the conference from these two churches amounted to less than $200,000 a year. Now there are six Adventist churches in the area with a total membership of about 2,500. The largest is the Kettering church about a block from the hospital, with just over 1,000 members. There are three* *new church buildings, and a 12-grade school in a modern building with about 350 students, instead of an 8-grade school with 41 students....*

"I close with a comment about a vital part of our health ministry and the final result we all strive for. It is the hope that the unpublicized, personal witness of the many individuals involved in bringing healing to the sick, combined with the public ministry of the word and song and service, will ultimately result in recognizing familiar but unexpected faces and hearing familiar but unexpected voices joining in the great song described in the colorful words of Revelation *15:3, 4."*

* Reprinted by permission, George Nelson, *The Kettering Medical Center: Recollections and Reflections on the Early Years*, 1996.

Appendix B

Chronology

The following list of hospitals and sanitariums that are or were operated by the Seventh-day Adventist church and/or one of the Adventist health systems was compiled while researching *A Thousand Miracles Every Day*. A few self-supporting facilities are also listed. In some cases the facilities did not operate continuously, and several of the dates are approximate. While not 100 percent complete, the list provides a fair record of the global presence of Adventist hospitals from 1866 to 2000.

YEAR(s)	HOSPITAL
1866–1908	Battle Creek Sanitarium, Battle Creek, Michigan
1878	St. Helena Hospital, Deer Park, California
1888–1912	Mount Vernon Sanitarium, Mount Vernon, Ohio
1893–1989	Boulder Memorial Hospital, Boulder, Colorado
1893–1905	Chicago Sanitarium, Chicago, Illinois
1893	Portland Adventist Medical Center, Portland, Oregon
1894–1907	Guadalajara Sanitarium, Mexico
1895	Lake Geneva Sanitarium, Switzerland
1895–1920	Nebraska Sanitarium, Lincoln, Nebraska
1895–1906	Samoa Sanitarium, Samoa
1897–1905	Claremont Sanitarium, South Africa
1898–1992	Skodsborg Sanitarium, Denmark
1899–1903	Avondale Health Retreat, Australia
1899–1999	Boston Regional Medical Center, Stoneham, Massachusetts
1899–1943	Iowa Sanitarium, Nevada, Iowa
1899	Walla Walla General Hospital, Walla Walla, Washington
1900–1907	Calcutta Sanitarium, India
1900–1912	Christchurch Sanitarium, New Zealand
1900–1906	Little Rock Sanitarium, Little Rock, Arkansas
1901–1924	Friedensau Sanitarium, Germany
1902–1907	Buffalo Sanitarium, Buffalo, New York
1902–1928	Kansas Sanitarium and Hospital, Wichita, Kansas
1902–1907	Keene Sanitarium (Lone Star Sanitarium), Keene, Texas
1902–1922	Madison Sanitarium, Madison, Wisconsin
1902–1924	Tri-City Sanitarium, Moline, Illinois
1903–1906	Arizona Sanitarium, Phoenix, Arizona

1903–	Atlanta Sanitarium, Atlanta, Georgia
1903–1949	Dr. Harry Miller's arrival marks the beginning of Adventist sanitariums and clinics in China. According to the 1951 *Yearbook*, more than a dozen facilities were operating in 1949.
1903–1908	Knowlton Sanitarium, Canada
1903–1922	Madison Sanitarium, Madison, Wisconsin
1903	Sydney Adventist Hospital, Australia
1904–1934	Cape Sanitarium, South Africa
1904–1915	Graysville Sanitarium and Hospital, Graysville, Tennessee
1904	Paradise Valley Hospital, National City, California
1904–	Philadelphia Sanitarium, Philadelphia, Pennsylvania
1905	Glendale Adventist Medical Center, Glendale, California
1905–1980s	Gopalganj Hospital, Bangladesh
1905	Loma Linda University Medical Center, Loma Linda, California
1905	Hinsdale Hospital, Hinsdale, Illinois
1905–1997	Nyhyttan Health and Rehabilitation Center, Sweden
1906–1932	Wabash Valley Sanitarium, Lafayette, Indiana
1907–1913	Black River Sanitarium, Watertown, New York
1907	Tennessee Christian Medical Center Portland, Portland, Tennessee
1907	Washington Adventist Hospital, Takoma Park, Maryland
1908–1919	Adelaide Sanitarium, Australia
1908	Florida Hospital, Orlando, Florida
1908	Malamulo Hospital, Malawi
1908–1910	Mussoorie Sanitarium, India
1908–1927	Nebraska Branch Sanitarium, Hastings, Nebraska
1908	River Plate Sanitarium and Hospital, Argentina
1908-WW II	Soonan Hospital, Korea
1908	Tennessee Christian Medical Center, Madison, Tennessee
1909–1912	Rock City Sanitarium, Nashville, Tennessee
1910–1923	Huntsville Sanitarium, Huntsville, Alabama
1910	Park Ridge Hospital, Fletcher, North Carolina
1910–2000	Warburton Adventist Hospital, Australia
1912–1968	Stanboroughs Nursing and Maternity Home, England
1913	White Memorial Medical Center, Los Angeles, California
1914–1992	Hadley Memorial Hospital, Washington, D.C.
1914–1988	Scott Memorial Hospital, Lawrenceburg, Tennessee
1915–1949	Nanning Seventh-day Adventist Hospital, China
1915	Simla Sanitarium and Hospital, India
1916–1968	Chuharkana Hospital Dispensary, Pakistan
1916–1947	Yencheng Sanitarium, China

1917–1925	Bethel Sanitarium, Canada
1918–1923	Douglasville Sanitarium, Douglasville, Georgia
1918–1949	Shanghai Medical Center, China
1920	Berlin Hospital, Germany
1920–	El Reposo Sanitarium, Florence, Alabama
1920–1957	Pisgah Sanitarium and Hospital, Candler, North Carolina
1921	Kanye Hospital, Botswana
1921–1979	Rest Haven Hospital, Canada
1922	Juliaca Adventist Clinic, Peru
1924	Penang Adventist Hospital, Malaysia
1925	Giffard Memorial Hospital, India
1925	Kendu Adventist Hospital, Kenya
1925-WW II	Narsapur Seventh–day Adventist Mission Hospital, India
1925–	Pewee Valley Sanitarium, near Louisville, Kentucky
1926	Hultafors Health Centre, Sweden
1927–1958	Georgia Sanitarium, Atlanta, Georgia
1927	Mwami Adventist Hospital, Zambia
1927–1983	Riverside Sanitarium and Hospital, Nashville, Tennessee
1927	Songa Adventist Hospital, Democratic Republic of Congo
1928–1975	Bongo Mission Hospital, Angola
1928–1977	Sonnenhof Sanitarium, Germany
1928	Takoma Adventist Hospital, Greeneville, Tennessee
1929	Manila Sanitarium and Hospital, Philippines
1929–1936, 1953–1974	Taffari Makonnen Hospital, Ethiopia
1929	Tokyo Adventist Hospital, Japan
1930	Porter Adventist Hospital, Denver, Colorado
1930–1939	Sultanbad Hospital, Iran
1931	Mugonero Hospital, Rwanda
1932–1976	Empress Zauditu Memorial Adventist Hospital, Ethiopia
1934–1975	Haile Selassie I Hospital, Ethiopia
1934–1991	Pine Forest Sanitarium and Hospital, Gilbertown, Alabama
1935–	Lanchow Sanitarium, China
1935	Seoul Adventist Hospital, Korea
1936–1978	Kwailibesi Hospital, Solomon Islands
1936–1959	Nokuphila Hospital, South Africa
1936	Surat Hospital, India
1936–1949	Wuhan Sanitarium, China
1937	Bangkok Adventist Hospital, Thailand
1937–1995	Fuller Memorial Hospital, South Attleboro, Massachusetts
1937–1978	Kukudu Hospital (Amyes Memorial Hospital), Solomon Islands
1937–1945	Maun Medical Mission Hospital, Zambesi

1939–1942	Good View Clinic, Brazil
1940	Little Creek Sanitarium, Knoxville, Tennessee
1940	Phuket Adventist Hospital, Thailand
1942	Sao Paulo Adventist Hospital, Brazil
1942	Wildwood Sanitarium, Wildwood, Georgia
1943	Hopeaniemi Health and Rehabilitation Center, Finland
1944	Seventh-day Adventist Hospital Ile-Ife, Nigeria
1945	Andrews Memorial Hospital, Jamaica, West Indies
1946–1959	Dar Es-Salaam Hospital, aka The House of Peace Hospital, Iraq
1946	Miraflores Adventist Clinic, Peru
1946	Montemorelos University Hospital, Mexico
1946	Skogli Health and Rehabilitation Center, Norway
1947–1992	Ardmore Adventist Hospital, Ardmore, Oklahoma
1947–1964	Forsyth Memorial Sanitarium and Hospital, Tallahassee, Florida
1947	Gimbie Hospital, Ethiopia
1947	Jengre Seventh-day Adventist Hospital, Nigeria
1947–1965	Rangoon Adventist Hospital, Myanmar (Burma)
1948	Community Hospital of Seventh-day Adventists, Trinidad, West Indies
1948	Florida Hospital Heartland Medical Center, Sebring, Florida (formerly Walker Memorial Hospital, Avon Park)
1948–1980	Nicaragua Adventist Hospital, Nicaragua
1948	Silvestre Adventist Hospital, Brazil
1948–1995	Youngberg Memorial Adventist Hospital, Singapore
1949	Heri Adventist Hospital, Tanzania
1949	Ranchi Adventist Hospital, India
1950	Bandung Adventist Hospital, Java, Indonesia
1950	Feather River Hospital, Paradise, California
1950	Ishaka Adventist Hospital, Uganda
1950	Karachi Adventist Hospital, Pakistan
1950	Penfigo Adventist Hospital, Brazil
1950–1982	Togoba Hospital, New Guinea
1951	Maluti Adventist Hospital, South Africa
1951	Pusan Adventist Hospital, Korea
1952	Mindanao Sanitarium and Hospital, Philippines
1952	North Norway Rehabilitation Center, Norway
1952	Penfigo Adventist Hospital, Brazil
1953	Adventist Medical Center, Okinawa, Japan
1953	Belem Adventist Hospital, Brazil
1954	Bella Vista Hospital, Puerto Rico
1954	Davis Memorial Clinic and Hospital, Guyana

1954–1988	Haad Yai Mission Hospital, Thailand
1954–1964	Iceland Summer Sanitarium, Iceland
1954	Koza Adventist Hospital, Republic of Cameroon
1955–1978	Boliu Hospital, Papua New Guinea
1955–1974	Kwahu Hospital, Ghana
1955–1975	Saigon Adventist Hospital, Vietnam
1955–1970	Santa Ana Hospital, Santa Anna, Texas
1955	Taiwan Adventist Hospital, Taiwan
1955	Yuka Adventist Hospital, Zambia
1956–1969	Benghazi Adventist Hospital, Libya
1956	Guam Seventh-day Adventist Clinic, Guam
1956	H. W. Miller Memorial Sanitarium and Hospital, Philippines
1957	Blantyre Adventist Hospital, Malawi
1957–1997	North York Branson Hospital, Canada
1957	Sonora Community Hospital, Sonora, California
1957–1980	Watkins Memorial Hospital, Ellijay, Georgia
1958–1992	Louis Smith Memorial Hospital, Lakeland, Georgia
1958–1980	Menard Hospital, Menard, Texas
1958–1972	Putnam Memorial Hospital, Palatka, Florida
1959	Asuncion Adventist Sanitarium, Paraguay
1959	Belgrano Adventist Clinic, Argentina
1959	Cagayan Valley Sanitarium and Hospital, Philippines
1959–1992	Parkview Memorial Hospital, Brunswick, Maine
1960	Central Texas Medical Center, San Marcos, Texas
1960–	Reading Rehabilitation Hospital, Reading, Pennsylvania
1960	Scheer Memorial Hospital, Nepal
1961	Ana Stahl Adventist Clinic, Peru
1961–1996	Monument Valley Hospital, Mexican Hat, Utah
1961–1970s	New Hebrides SDA Mission Hospital, New Hebrides
1961	Quito Adventist Clinic, Ecuador
1961	Sopas Adventist Hospital, Papua New Guinea
1961–1981	Tempe Community Hospital, Tempe, Arizona
1962	Gingoog Sanitarium and Hospital, Philippines
1962–1985	Memorial Hospital of Bee County, Beeville, Texas
1962	Shawnee Mission Medical Center, Shawnee Mission, Kansas
1963	Castle Medical Center, Kailua, Hawaii
1963	Hanford Community Medical Center, Hanford, California
1964	Kettering Medical Center, Kettering, Ohio
1964	San Joaquin Community Hospital
1964	Tsuen Wan Adventist Hospital, Hong Kong
1965	Bacolod Sanitarium and Hospital, Philippines
1965	Hohenau Adventist Sanitarium, Paraguay

1965–1985	Jay Memorial Hospital, Jay, Oklahoma
1965	Lakeside Adventist Hospital, Sri Lanka
1965	Masanga Leprosy Hospital, Sierra Leone
1965	Simi Valley Hospital and Health Care Services, Simi Valley, California
1966	Atoifi Adventist Hospital, Solomon Islands
1966–1978	Kastiorita Hospital, Papua New Guinea
1966	Loma Linda Adventist Sanitarium, Argentina
1966	Roundelwood (Good Health Association), Scotland
1966	Ruby Nelson Memorial Hospital, India
1969–1986	Marion County Hospital, Jefferson, Texas
1969	Medan Adventist Hospital, Indonesia
1969–1994	Medical Center Hospital, Punta Gorda, Florida
1969	Ottapalam Seventh-day Adventist Hospital, India
1970	Antillean Adventist Hospital, Curacao, Netherlands Antilles
1970	Cave Memorial Clinic and Nursing Home, Barbados, West Indies
1971	Hongkong Adventist Hospital, Hong Kong
1971	Memorial Hospital, Manchester, Kentucky
1972	Northeast Argentine Sanitarium, Argentina
1973	Calbayog Sanitarium and Hospital, Philippines
1973	Florida Hospital Altamonte, Altamonte Springs, Florida
1973	Hackettstown Community Hospital, Hackettstown, New Jersey
1973	Kobe Adventist Hospital, Japan
1973	Tillamook County General Hospital, Tillamook, Oregon
1973–	Toole County Adventist Hospital, Shelby, Montana
1974–2000	Auckland Adventist Hospital, New Zealand
1974	Jellico Community Hospital, Jellico, Tennessee
1974	Pune Adventist Hospital, India
1974	Valley of the Angels Hospital, Honduras
1975–1991	Anacapa Adventist Hospital, Port Hueneme, California
1975	Florida Hospital Apopka, Apopka, Florida
1975	Southeast Hospital, Mexico
1976	Andapa Adventist Hospital, Madagascar
1976	Emory Adventist Hospital, Smyrna, Georgia
1977	Huguley Memorial Medical Center, Fort Worth, Texas
1978	Adventist Hospital of Haiti, Haiti
1978	Bangalore Adventist Hospital, India
1978	Manaus Adventist Hospital, Brazil
1979	Shady Grove Adventist Hospital, Rockville, Maryland
1979	Ukiah Valley Medical Center, Ukiah, California
1980	Chippewa Valley Hospital, Durand, Wisconsin

1980	Sao Roque Adventist Clinic, Brazil
1981	Gordon Hospital, Calhoun, Georgia
1982	Espirito Santo Adventist Hospital, Brazil
1982	Florida Hospital Lake Placid, Lake Placid, Florida
1982	LaPaz Adventist Clinic, Bolivia
1982	Palawan Adventist Hospital, Philippines
1982–1994	Moberly Regional Medical Center, Moberly, Missouri
1982–1987	Reeves County Hospital, Pecos, Texas
1983	Los Angeles Adventist Clinic, Chile
1982–1988	Sierra Vista Hospital, Truth or Consequences, New Mexico
1983	Metroplex Hospital, Killeen, Texas
1983	Venezuela Adventist Hospital, Venezuela
1984	Asamang Seventh-day Adventist Hospital, Ghana
1984	Milton Mattison Memorial Hospital, India
1984	Seventh-day Adventist Hospital and Motherless Babies' Home, Nigeria
1985	East Pasco Medical Center, Zephyrhills, Florida
1986	Seventh-day Adventist Cooper Hospital, Liberia
1987	Davao Sanitarium and Hospital, Philippines
1987	San Joaquin Community Hospital, Bakersfield, California
1989	Avista Adventist Hospital, Louisville, Colorado
1989	Littleton Adventist Hospital, Littleton, Colorado
1989	Porto Alegre Adventist Clinic, Brazil
1990s	Glei Adventist Eye Hospital, Togo
1990	Bella Vista Polyclinic, Puerto Rico
1990	Dominase Adventist Hospital, Ghana
1990	Florida Hospital East Orlando, Orlando, Florida
1991	Batouri Adventist Hospital, Republic of Cameroon
1991	Rollins-Brook Community Hospital, Lampasas, Texas
1992	Florida Hospital Waterman, Eustis, Florida
1993	Florida Hospital Kissimmee, Kissimmee, Florida
1993	Florida Hospital Wauchula, Wauchula, Florida
1994	Bandar Lampung Adventist Hospital, Sumatra, Indonesia
1994	East Bolivia Adventist Clinic, Bolivia
1994	Florida Hospital Fish Memorial, Orange City, Florida
1996	Aizawl Adventist Hospital, India
1996	Thanjavur Adventist Hospital, India
1997	Florida Hospital Celebration Health, Celebration, Florida
1997	GlenOaks Medical Center, Glendale Heights, Illinois
1997	Nova Friburgo Adventist Hospital, Brazil
1998	Southern Medical Center, Puerto Rico
1999	La Grange Memorial Hospital, La Grange, Illinois

2000	Memorial Hospital-Flagler, Bunnell, Florida
2000	Memorial Hospital-Ormond Beach, Ormond Beach, Florida
2000	Memorial Hospital-Peninsula, Ormond Beach, Florida
2000	Florida Hospital Deland, Deland, Florida
2000	Winter Park Memorial Hospital, Winter Park, Florida